LIVING WITH ENDOMETRIOSIS

The Complete Guide to Risk Factors,
Symptoms, and Treatment Options

Samantha Bowick

Foreword by Ken Sinervo, MD

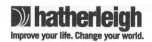

hatherleigh
Improve your life. Change your world.

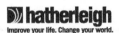

Improve your life. Change your world.

Hatherleigh Press is committed to preserving and protecting the natural resources of the earth. Environmentally responsible and sustainable practices are embraced within the company's mission statement.

Visit us at www.hatherleighpress.com and register online for free offers, discounts, special events, and more.

Living with Endometriosis
Text copyright © 2018 Samantha Bowick

Library of Congress Cataloging-in-Publication Data is available upon request.
ISBN: 978-1-57826-746-0

Interior Design by Cynthia Dunne

Printed in the United States
10 9 8 7 6 5 4

CONTENTS

For all of my "Endo Sisters."

And thank you to everyone who has been there for me. I do not know what I would have done without all of your help and support through-out this difficult time in my life.

AUTHOR'S NOTE

I am not a doctor, nor do I claim to be. I am not suggesting you try a specific treatment outlined in this book; I am providing you with treatment options and what worked for me. However, just because something worked for me does not mean it will work for you; likewise, just because a treatment did *not* work for me does not mean it will not work for you.

I have written my story in hopes that it will help someone suffering with endometriosis make the best decision for their body.

AN OPEN LETTER TO ENDOMETRIOSIS

Dear Endometriosis,

You have caused me so much pain and heartache that I do not even know where to begin. The only thing I hate in this world is you. How can you come and go as you please and make women suffer so much pain? You keep me up at night with your pain, headaches, and nausea. Because of you, I have had to put my dreams, my life on hold. You have even forced me to have a hysterectomy; I hope you are happy.

But we *will* find a cure, sooner rather than later. And when we do, you better watch out! You have ruined my life for so many years, but for me, it stops now!

> Signed,
> A Strong Endo Warrior

FOREWORD

I F YOU have ever experienced pelvic pain, you are not alone. Although it can be difficult to talk about, in *Living with Endometriosis,* Samantha has bravely shared her long journey in this moving and inspirational book in the hopes that others may learn from her experiences and connect with important resources to live full, vibrant lives in spite of their condition.

Affecting an estimated 176 million individuals globally, from every ethnic and social background, endometriosis is commonly characterized by pelvic pain (which may become chronic over time), organ dysfunction, debilitating menstrual pain, infertility/pregnancy loss, and painful sex (dyspareunia). Typically affecting the pelvic region, endometriosis may also uncommonly present in such remote locations as the lungs. Although it is among the most prevalent of diseases, this enigmatic condition remains poorly understood and is responsible for billions of dollars annually in healthcare, lost productivity, and indirect costs.

The effects of endometriosis, which may also be linked to certain other health concerns and gynepathologies, can be systemic in nature and are much larger than just "painful periods." The condition has the capacity to significantly impair every aspect of an affected individual's life, from physical, sexual, and emotional health to career and academic opportunities. Yet despite its far-reaching impact, symptoms are often mistakenly normalized as "a part of womanhood," particularly in adolescence, when the disease may first present. Such persistent myths and misinformation continue to enshroud the disorder, resulting in long diagnostic delays, poor information systems, and continued ineffective care and support of those suffering.

Unfortunately, due to the vast inaccuracies surrounding the disease, it remains difficult for some patients to get quality care for endometriosis, despite its staggering personal and societal impact. Many individuals seeking answers may be told their symptoms are "in their head," or have their pain simply blamed on "bad cramps," resulting in barriers to quality care and an average ten-year delay in diagnosis. However, endometriosis pain is not "in your head," and "bad cramps" don't keep a person out of work or school; symptoms like chronic pelvic pain, painful intercourse, debilitating periods, backache, and painful bowel and bladder symptoms, on the other hand, are very suggestive of the condition.

Even in cases of timely diagnosis, an individual with endometriosis may struggle with poor care and experience frustration at the lack of dialogue with their physicians, side effects of treatments, and limited access to all the options that exist. They may only be offered ineffective (and potentially harmful) drug therapies that merely quell symptoms on a temporary basis, incomplete surgery that leaves disease behind, or may even be counseled to undergo a potentially unnecessary hysterectomy under the guise of a cure (which it is not). They may also be told that pregnancy or menopause will cure them—untrue and painful advice for someone with endometriosis-related infertility. Left inadequately treated, the disease can lead to continued or worsening pain, infertility or pregnancy loss, anatomic dysfunction, and the associated costs that contribute to the high financial, physical, and intangible burdens of endometriosis.

Unfortunately, as doctors we are trained early on to believe that there is no difference in how endometriosis is treated—but in reality, there is an excess of evidence to support Laparoscopic Excision (LAPEX) over incomplete disease removal. Patients with endometriosis can benefit from excision as the surgical cornerstone of a high-quality, multidisciplinary treatment plan, allowing for endometriosis and other causes of pelvic pain to be addressed, both during surgery and post-operatively through important adjuncts like pelvic floor therapy. LAPEX offers a significant improvement in sexual functioning, quality of life, and pain levels, while on the other hand, superficial removal—commonly performed outside of specialty centers—simply destroys tissue, making microscopic evaluation impossible and leaving disease behind, leading to persistent symptoms. However, the most important thing when planning a patient's treatment for endometriosis, above all else, is to listen to them.

The most critical step towards long-term, successful management of endometriosis is early diagnosis. Recognizing symptoms and getting effective help and treatment at the first signs can help prevent a vicious cycle of years of severe disease, misdiagnosis, progressive symptoms, and failed treatments. Finding a physician who is truly educated about endometriosis and understands your pain may be difficult, but they do exist. Help is out there. Believe in yourself; if you think you have endometriosis, seek the advice of true experts and become a partner in your care. Pursue early diagnosis and effective intervention through LAPEX and multidisciplinary care if at all possible. Use your voice and tell your story, as Samantha has.

Don't be discouraged by this disease—you are strong and you can get through it. We can almost always win the battle … together.

—Ken Sinervo, MD, MSc, FRCSC, ACGE, Medical Director, Center for Endometriosis Care, 2017–2018 Chairman, Endometriosis & Reproductive Surgery Special Interest Group, AAGL

INTRODUCTION

I AM NOT telling my story so that people will feel sorry for me; I want them to understand, as best as they can, just how much pain we go through on a daily basis and how much our lives change because of endometriosis.

Let me start off by saying that you are not alone and that you *will* get through this. Over the years, I have done an extensive amount of research on pelvic pain and endometriosis (one of the many benefits of having a smartphone while sitting in waiting rooms) to better educate myself. I knew when I first started having pain there was something wrong; my body would not be hurting if everything was fine, right? It is not normal to be in pain at all, whether it be pelvic pain or any other type of pain. If you are in pain, it is time to get help.

Any woman can have endometriosis. A woman may have the disease and her sister may also have it, but not show any symptoms; it depends on the person. There are even celebrities who struggle with endometriosis. But you'd never know to look at them; those of us with endometriosis are forced to be the strongest women we can be, doing as much as possible to hide how much pain we are really in. Having been through so much physical pain, we can handle anything that comes our way!

But because we do not want people to pity or feel sorry for us, we instead put on a happy face and smile through the pain. Perhaps you feel that if you were to talk about it with someone, they would brush it off, saying it is all in your head. I have had quite a few doctors tell me just that, and it is extremely upsetting every time it happens.

But I just kept pushing, seeking the answers I so desperately needed. And now, I am so thankful I had the willpower to do that.

Nobody wants to talk about female problems, but not talking about them does nothing to help anyone—and that is where I draw the line. I am going to share every aspect of my journey—the good, the bad, and the ugly—in the hopes that it will help you live a healthier life sooner, rather than later. Hopefully, my story will inspire you to seek the help that you need to live the healthy, pain-free life you so deserve. Remember: it is not your fault you are in pain; it is not anyone's fault. While it may be hard to find a doctor out there who really cares and who knows what they are talking about, just keep fighting, because they *are* out there.

WHAT IS ENDOMETRIOSIS?

The endometrium is the lining of the uterus that sheds every month during what's known as your period. Endometriosis is a condition where tissue similar to the lining of the uterus (the endometrial stroma and glands, which should only be located inside the uterus) is found elsewhere in the body[1]. Places this disease can be found include (but are not limited to): colon, rectum, appendix, ovaries, and fallopian tubes. Some women may have endometriosis on many organs in their body, but may not experience any pain, while others may have a small amount of disease, but excruciating pain.

If a woman has endometriosis, when it is "that time of the month" the endometriosis tissue that is on the other organs—for example, the ovaries—will also bleed just as the normal tissue does. This causes inflammation, which causes pain. It is

---

1   endometriosis.org/endometriosis

not known why this happens, or why it is more painful in some women than in others, but it is known that estrogen causes the endometriosis to continue growing.

Some of the symptoms of endometriosis include pelvic pain, painful periods (cramping), infertility, and pain during sexual intercourse. Sometimes, other conditions can be confused with endometriosis; for me, my misdiagnosis was irritable bowel syndrome. This type of misdiagnosis means it takes the patient longer to be properly diagnosed with endometriosis and receive treatment.

While reading, keep in mind that everyone is different, so what works for me may not work for you, and vice versa. By no means do I claim to be a doctor. I have been through the agonizing pain of endometriosis for many years and have experienced the treatments available for endometriosis, which is what I look to write about here.

I missed out on so many fun things because of this disease. I am now twenty-seven years old, and most people my age are out partying, taking trips, or enjoying college. But I could not do any of the things I enjoyed because I knew I would be in constant pain. I have felt like a lot of people do not see me as a person after they hear about my diagnosis. Instead, they see me as my diagnosis: endometriosis.

This book presents my experiences with endometriosis in the order that they took place in my life. I hope by writing all of this, I can help more women understand this disease, and perhaps help doctors to understand how their patients suffering with this awful disease really feel.

1

My Story

I REMEMBER THE first time I started my period like it was yesterday, just as every woman does. I was thirteen, on my way back from vacation visiting family with my father and sister, and we stopped off to get something to eat. When I went to the bathroom and saw I had started, I began silently freaking out, but I did not let anyone know I'd started until we got home. At the time, I thought it was the greatest day of my life. I was eager to be a woman and an adult, just as every child is.

Little did I know that I would soon get a rude awakening.

The pain began when I started my period, but at first, I only had pain during my periods. It wasn't until I graduated high school and started college that the pain became more severe. My ovaries would hurt even when I was not on my period, and I was already on birth control to help control menstrual cramps and heavy bleeding. At the beginning, taking baths or using a heating pad would decrease the amount of pain I was in. But the older I got, the less those remedies helped--most likely because my body was so accustomed to being in constant pain. But all people would tell me was to "take a Midol" for the pain, which only infuriated me. They seemed unwilling to understand that I was not just having period cramps.

As I got older, it became harder for me to wear tampons,

to the point that I just chose not to wear them. Once, in 8th grade, I decided to wear a super-sized tampon to school—a huge mistake. I did not realize how much I was bleeding, and blood got on my clothes, meaning I had to call home. In a matter of two hours, my tampon needed to be changed because I was bleeding so much. I never let that happen again! But when I told my doctor about this, she did not think anything of it.

I could always tell when it was "that time of the month" by the way I felt. My stomach would hurt and I would feel nauseous to the point where I did not want to eat anything. This caused me to miss so much school and, as I got older, work. While in pain, I never once had a friend offer to come over and sit with me, at least for the first few years of my diagnosis. Not once did they say, "Hey, would you like for me to come over and watch a movie with you, or bring you something?" I do not know if it was because they thought I did not want to be bothered, if they did not care, or did not believe I was really in pain.

Every female in my family had or has cramps, so they brushed it off and told me it was normal—just a part of growing up. My first encounter with endometriosis was around age fifteen, when I heard how a cousin (on my dad's side of the family) was going to have laparoscopic surgery to remove her endometriosis. A few years after having two children, my cousin ended up having a hysterectomy because she was in so much pain, but to no avail; her pain continued. A few years after that, I began having the same problems she did.

I have spent so many days and nights lying in bed, crying, frustrated with the medical community because (up until recently) I was getting absolutely no help. I was angry that I was in pain and could not work or go to school. I felt so alone because hardly anyone around me understood what I was going through. I hardly had any friends I could count on to be there when I needed them. It is a pain I would not wish on anyone.

MY SYMPTOMS

Starting at a young age, I had horrible cramps, as well as head-aches, around the time of each of my periods. However, as time went on, both the pelvic pain and headaches became constant. I had trouble sleeping, which led to me feeling fatigued and having no energy. It was hard to focus because of the constant pain, and it became a battle for me to even get out of bed every day. Pelvic exams caused excruciating pain, which led to me not wanting to go to the doctor. It is even possible to bleed af-ter pelvic exams, which occurred with me many times. I always felt nauseous and could not pinpoint the reason. I felt like my insides were literally going to fall out onto the floor.

Doctors did not take me seriously when I told them this. But that was the only way I felt I could accurately describe the pain. Instead, doctors would put me through yet another painful pelvic exam and would find nothing wrong. Then they would do an ultrasound, which invariably showed at least one cyst on one of my ovaries.

All I wanted was someone to listen to me and let me vent, cry on their shoulder, or whatever I felt like doing. Instead, I received countless opinions about what I should be doing or how I could better "cope." So many people told me that I was too young to have so many problems. Believe me, I agreed with them, but that didn't make my pain any less real.

MY DOCTORS

In the course of my treatment for endometriosis, I have been to a total of thirty-one medical professionals (as of this publication). This number includes a variety of doctors, including gynecolo-gists, a urologist, gastroenterologists, a woman's health specialist that specializes in bio-identical hormones, a physical therapist, endometriosis specialists, endocrinologists, and a rheumatologist.

The first gynecologist I went to was in 2009. I explained my symptoms of "cramping," and she wrote me a prescription for Ortho Tri-cyclen Lo, a birth control pill, and told me I was to follow the instructions on the pack, which I did. I took the pill and, not feeling any pain relief, went back for a follow-up appointment and had an ultrasound, which is how the gynecologist found a cyst on my right ovary.

We decided that I needed to have surgery, and she performed a laparoscopic procedure on me in July 2010, on my father's 50th birthday of all days. My parents and I were told after the fact that the doctor had drained the cyst and found something that looked like endometriosis, so she cauterized it, which is burning the disease (this method can lead to scarring). However, she did not send what she found off for testing.

At the time, I knew very little about this disease, and the doctor did little to explain it. I remember feeling so lost and confused, a situation that would soon become all too familiar. This is indicative of the wider experience endometriosis sufferers tend to have with their medical practitioners; a combination of ignorance and misinformation on both sides. For example, I now know that cauterizing is not the best way to get rid of endometriosis—something I wish I'd known at the time. I would ask each doctor if I should be in this much pain during and after a pelvic exam. Their responses ranged from yes (because I was a virgin) to "no, but I am not sure why it is so painful for you."

This ignorance is frustrating but hardly surprising. Doctors go to school for several years yet know absolutely nothing about endometriosis because it is not in most textbooks, and if it is in their textbooks, the information is not the most accurate.

After my first surgery, I told my doctor that I was still in pain. Her response nearly floored me: she explained that I should not be in pain anymore and that, if I was, there was nothing else she could do for me. She suggested that I get pregnant; that would make the pain go away. I understand the reasoning; if I was pregnant, I would not have a period. Because of this, my endometrium would not shed and any endometriosis would not grow. But this didn't guarantee that I'd be pain-free after pregnancy, if I became pregnant. However, I thought then (and still believe now) that having a child should be my decision, not my doctor's. At this point in my life, I wanted to have children, but was not ready to have any yet. I wanted to graduate college first, and then get married. So, as politely as I could, I explained that I was not ready to become pregnant, and switched doctors as soon as I could.

After my first laparoscopic surgery, I switched to another gynecologist. She tried different treatments, but soon she was all out of ideas and just left me twisting in the wind. Her focus was a battery of birth control medications. Working with her, I tried everything from Necon to Seasonique to Lupron injections. None of the birth control pills helped my pain, though the Lupron helped a little bit.

Since I was still not getting the kind of pain relief she thought I should, she decided to refer me to a local gastroenterologist, who performed a CT scan and a colonoscopy and diagnosed me with irritable bowel syndrome. I took the medicine he prescribed (Hyoscyamine) for almost a year, but my pain was not relieved. The gynecologist ended up performing another laparoscopic surgery in 2012, after which I was told that she had drained another cyst on my right ovary and that she did not see any evidence that I had *ever* had endometriosis.

Two months after the surgery, I had a period that lasted for three weeks. I went to the emergency room where they told me to call my doctor. I did as they asked and left a voicemail for her to call me, but she never did. On to the next doctor, then.

For a time, I tried to do without doctors (who didn't seem to have any answers for me anyway), and worked to manage my symptoms on my own. I became very depressed because I was in so much pain and had so many conflicting diagnoses.

I was accepted into pharmacy school, but had to quit. I moved out from my parents' home for a month, to a place of my own about two hours away, but that did not work because I was in too much pain to function, much less study and do all the things I needed to.

After I quit pharmacy school, I also quit my job at a local pharmacy. I was unemployed for almost seven months when I decided I'd had enough of endometriosis ruining my life. I applied for a job at an independent pharmacy, and by the grace of God, I was hired. I am so thankful I was employed there; at the time, I had no idea just how harmful birth control pills are to women, or that there are other approaches that can be used to diminish pelvic pain.

I began visiting doctors again, starting with a urologist who performed Magnetic Resonance Imaging (MRI) and some bladder tests to see if I had interstitial cystitis (discussed more in Chapter 8). At this point, I was told there was nothing wrong with my bladder, but that it was good for that to be ruled out. However, I *did* have free fluid in my pelvis, something which my urologist never told me. I only found out when I printed my results online. (Most of the time, free fluid is not a big deal, but it my case it *could* be, and the doctor should have made a point to tell me.)

I even went to a fertility doctor, but he could not help with the pain, either. He thought if I took a birth control pill with add-back therapy, it would help my symptoms. Unfortunately, it just made things worse.

At this time, I felt ready to find an endometriosis specialist to perform another surgery. I began trying to find doctors on-line that were close to my area, until I found one about three hours away from me who seemed to be a great endometriosis specialist. In 2013, a year after the last surgery, I went under the knife again. The doctor performing this surgery used a differ-ent technique to remove the endometriosis; he also removed my appendix, since it is not needed and he wanted to make sure I would not have endometriosis grow on it. He found the disease in my colon and rectum, as well as in my pelvic wall. He ruled that I was a stage I case of endometriosis--however, the stage of one's disease does not determine how painful the disease is; it only denotes how much disease is found in the body.

After the surgery, he recommended having a Mirena put in—an intrauterine device (IUD). After doing research and seeing commercials for malpractice suits against similar devices, I decided I did not want to have the intrauterine device in my body. There was too much research that suggests it can migrate from where it is supposed to be. After I refused the IUD, he told me there weren't any other options besides a hysterectomy, so I was once again in search of a new doctor—one who would listen to me. After all, a hysterectomy could never be anything but a last resort for me; I still wanted to have kids when I was ready.

In my seemingly endless search for answers, I even signed up for a violet petal study in hopes of some pain relief. The violet petal study is a research study that looks to try and find a cure for endometriosis. Unfortunately, I could not participate because I still had the last dose of Lupron in my system. Doctors do this study in many areas, so if you are interested you may want to look it up online and request more information. Just remember that the researchers do not know much about the medications being studied. Because of that, there could be adverse reactions they do not know about.

MY LAPAROSCOPIC SURGERIES

I'd like to go into a bit more detail about my experiences with laparoscopic surgery. My first laparoscopic surgery, in 2009, was not as bad as I thought it was going to be. I had two incisions: one at my belly button and the other on my right bikini line. However, I also feel like my doctor did not do much while she was operating. She drained a cyst and cauterized the area, but that was about it. I did have some trouble recovering, though, because I was unable to void on my own. I was taking college summer classes at the time, and I remember being in so much pain while at school because I could not go to the bathroom. After class I had to go to the doctor so she could catheterize me, which was terrible!

My second surgery, about a year and a half later, went about the same as the first. It was performed by a different doctor, but she made the same two incisions that my first doctor did and drained a cyst on my right ovary. However, she said she could not see anything wrong that would make her think I had ever had endometriosis. I was unable to void on my own again, so I was forced to use catheters.

My third surgery was performed by yet another doctor, but he was an endometriosis specialist. He used four incisions: one at my belly button, one at my bladder, and one on either side at my bikini line. I also had my appendix removed during this surgery. I remember worrying about how my incisions would look once they healed, but they do not look bad. He did find endometriosis on my colon, which he removed, and drained a cyst on my right ovary. He also performed a hysteroscopy to make sure everything was okay with my uterus. I was unable to void by myself yet again after surgery and had to purchase some catheters on my own, since this doctor was out of town.

Before each surgery, as well as the abdominal CT scan and colonoscopy, I had to drink certain laxatives beforehand to "clean me out." Before my surgeries, it was magnesium citrate, which I had to drink the night before each procedure. About an hour before my CT scan, I had to drink a contrast, which was a white, chalky liquid that would allow my doctor to see my insides better on the x-ray.

THE LAST STRAW

As I have mentioned, I had to quit pharmacy school when I was twenty years old because my pain was so bad that it caused my grades to suffer. My dream—to one day own a pharmacy—seemed impossible. At the time, I was trying to make sense of it all. I believe everything happens for a reason, but the only reason I could come up with for everything that was happening to me was that I was somehow not meant to go to pharmacy school, even though that was all I wanted to do. The thought of this was devastating.

Meanwhile, my pain was reaching the point where I would have to pull my car over while driving because my pain was so bad. My insides felt like someone was squeezing and twisting them. One day, while sitting on the side of the road trying to hold my insides together, I called my doctor's office. Of course, it was a Friday and the office was "closed," and the nurse who answered told me I would have to wait until Monday to come in.

I was furious! I explained to her that I had to pull off at a gas station because my pain was so bad. She did not care. I was on my way to work, but once they found out what was going on, I was told not to come in. So instead of being seen by my doctor or getting my work done for the day, I went home to lie in my bed in pain.

It was then that I realized I had to do something about my health, and it needed to be done as soon as possible.

2

Endometriosis Explained

J UST WHAT *is* endometriosis?

Endometriosis is a debilitating disease surrounded by a lot of mystery, including about its exact causes and best methods of treatment. We know that endometriosis is primarily a disease that affects a woman's reproductive organs. However, the disease can be found in other parts of the body, including the heart, digestive tract, gallbladder, diaphragm, ovaries, uterus, and bladder. Unfortunately, there is no one known cause of the disease or one treatment that fits all who suffer with the agonizing pain and symptoms.

Some women who have endometriosis experience pain only around the time of their period, while others suffer with pain every day. Endometriosis is not just bad cramps; the way I have described it to people is the feeling of your insides twisting, barbed wire around you squeezing your waist, and feeling like your insides are going to fall out. None of these descriptions fit "bad cramps." Many people who don't have endometriosis can take Midol and their pain from cramping decreases or goes away. That is not the case for someone who suffers with endometriosis.

There are four stages of endometriosis: I, II, III, and IV. Stage I is the stage where very few endometrial implants are present, up

11

to stage IV, where the implants are more abundant. There could be so much disease present that organs could be bound to one another, which can cause a great deal of pain. Yet even though a woman may have only stage I endometriosis, she might experience more pain than a woman with stage IV. In short, the stage of one's endometriosis and amount of pain experienced do not have any correlation with one another.

It is important to note that not all cases of endometriosis are the same, and women who have the disease can experience different symptoms and may not display all of the known symptoms. Right now, it is known that estrogen feeds endometriosis. Many women who have the disease are estrogen dominant, which means the amount of estrogen their bodies have outweighs their amount of progesterone.

Symptoms of endometriosis include:

- Crippling period pain in menstruating females

- Abdominopelvic pain at any time, often intractable and chronic

- Bowel or urinary disorders/pain/dysfunction

- Painful intercourse/penetration/sexual activity

- Infertility/pregnancy loss and possible link to preterm births

- Immune-related and other comorbid disorders

- Allergies, migraines, or fatigue that may tend to worsen around menses

- Coughing up blood in cases of pleural/thoracic endometriosis

- Leg and lower back pain, particularly in cases of sciatic endometriosis

- The disease may also resemble some symptoms of, and has been linked to, adenomyosis (explained in Chapter 8)

- Data links chronic fatigue with menstrual abnormalities, endometriosis, pelvic pain, hysterectomy, and early/surgical menopause

- Comorbid pain syndromes, mood conditions, and asthma are also common in individuals with endometriosis

If you feel you have some of these symptoms, please be sure to talk to your doctor. It is better to be on the safe side and do something about it now.

The best treatment for endometriosis is laparoscopic surgery, a procedure in which the disease is excised. Laparoscopic surgery is done by going in through the patient's navel and possibly making other incisions on one of her sides, depending on how much endometriosis there is and how easy it is to remove (there are different ways to get rid of endometriosis, but the best way is by wide excision). However, laparoscopic surgery is not a cure; there is no definite known cause or cure for endometriosis at this time. Even though endometriosis can be removed, it can still come back in other places, or the surgeon could miss some of the disease, as it can sometimes be hard to find. Surgery can also cause scar tissue or adhesions, which are also painful.

Endometriosis is NOT in your head. I hope nobody has ever told you that or made you feel like this. If they have, know that you are not alone, and it is not in your head. There are medical treatments that may help you.

Samantha's Experience

When I first started experiencing pain, it was around the time I would be starting my period. I could always tell when it was that time because of how much pain I was in. I would try to plan as much of my life around when my period would be coming as much as possible, because I knew I would be laying in agony from pain and I didn't want to have to cancel plans unless I had to.

Once I graduated high school and started college, my pain level increased, as did the number of days I experienced pain. Before I had my first surgery, the number of days I experienced pain outnumbered my pain-free days. Then, every day I would experience some type of pain; some days were less painful than others, but the pain was always there, nagging. This interfered with my class attendance, grades, and work attendance. For my first two years of college, I took a full course load and worked part-time at a local pharmacy. While at school, I had to sit for hours at a time for classes and stand for hours for labs. While at work, I had to stand my entire shift, which was anywhere from four to six hours. This may not seem like much, but when you are already in pain, these long hours of staying in the same position only makes it worse.

GENETICS AND ENDOMETRIOSIS

Our genetic makeup plays a significant role in how our bodies react to different environmental stimuli, as well as what illnesses we are predisposed to or have a higher risk of developing. Endometriosis is among the diseases thought to have a genetic origin, though this connection is not fully understood; more research needs to be done to determine how much genetics influences endometriosis in different generations of families.

Samantha's Experience

Given my family history, I do believe that genetics plays a real role in endometriosis and how the disease progresses. On my dad's side of the family, I have one cousin who has been diagnosed with endometriosis. She was able to have two children before having a hysterectomy a few years after her second child was born. She's also had some of the same health issues that I have over the years. Her mother (my aunt) was diagnosed with PCOS, and has since passed away. Her daughter (my second cousin) is also thought to have endometriosis. Both my cousin and her daughter have experienced bowel issues similar to my own. My second cousin also had one of her fallopian tubes removed because it was swollen.

Meanwhile, my sister has recently been diagnosed with PCOS and has painful periods. Before being diagnosed, she had no reproductive issues that we knew of, but has been married for three years and has never been pregnant. My mother has had a cyst on one of her ovaries burst before, but has never been diagnosed with PCOS or endometriosis.

It seems quite possible that there is some genetic component to endometriosis, though whether it is a direct genetic cause or an underlying genetic aspect is subject to further study.

ENDOMETRIOSIS MYTHS

Other theories of causes of endometriosis include retrograde menstruation, immunologic dysfunction, homeobox genes, stem cells, and environmental toxins. There is no one correct or proven theory as of yet. There are, however, certain myths that surround the disease that I think anyone suffering with endometriosis needs to be aware of:

- A hysterectomy is not a cure for endometriosis; there is no known cure for the disease. A hysterectomy removes the organs, but not all of the disease.

- Getting pregnant is not a cure for endometriosis; neither is menopause. A pregnant woman will not have a period for nine months; however, after giving birth, she can experience endometriosis just as she did before.

- Shutting down the ovaries with medications prevents estrogen from being made, but it does not stop endometriosis from ever growing again.

- Women with endometriosis do not have the disease because they were sexually assaulted. The disease is not a sexually transmitted illness and is not caused from trauma.

- Abortion does not cause endometriosis.

- Teenagers can and do have endometriosis. The disease does not discriminate against age, race, or any other factors.

- Debilitating pain that interferes with your daily life is not normal. Again, endometriosis is *not* in your head.

Make sure to do your own endometriosis research before agreeing to any treatments and to discern fact from fiction. Make your decisions based on what you read and what you think is best for your body. It can be overwhelming, especially when you already feel horrible physically, but it is in your best interest. Sometimes, having endometriosis has felt like having a second job to me, with all of the doctor appointments I have went to and the amount of time I have put in trying to find a treatment that would work for my body. Don't give up; there is light at the end of the tunnel.

3

Surgical Treatment Options

I N THIS chapter, we'll review the different types of surgeries that are available for endometriosis treatment and how my body handled them.

Surgery is one of the more invasive treatments for endometriosis and remains controversial. Many gynecologists will operate on a patient without knowing much about the disease or what the best technique is to eradicate as much of the disease as possible. Unfortunately, only a handful of doctors in the United States use wide excision surgery when operating. This technique minimizes the risk of scar tissue in the future and the amount of disease left behind.

It is important that patients with endometriosis have as much information as possible to make the decision that is best for them. We'll discuss several surgical options in this chapter; for me, surgery helped me the most out of all of the treatments I tried, and I wish I'd known about wide excision surgery when I was first diagnosed. Any type of surgery is scary. Since surgeries often need to be scheduled months in advance, patients have plenty of time to sit and think about what's to come.

LAPAROSCOPIC SURGERY
Years ago, doctors used to perform surgeries by using bigger

incisions and opening the patient up. Now, doctors usually use laparoscopic surgery. Laparoscopic surgery is minimally invasive and is the most common type of surgery used for the treatment of endometriosis. The doctor makes small incisions (the number of incisions depends on where the doctor is looking and how much disease there is) which allows the surgeon to insert a camera as well as instruments to look around the pelvic region and any other possible areas that could have endometriosis. This is all done under general anesthesia, with the patient closely monitored from beginning to end.

The doctor will insert a catheter to empty the patient's bladder and will fill the patient's abdomen with CO_2 gas. This expands the patient's abdomen so that it is easier to see during surgery. The surgeon will look for disease, cysts, and any other abnormalities that could be present. The surgeon may then choose to stitch or glue the incisions during closing and cover them with gauze and/or bandages for them to heal. The patient will then be required to see the surgeon a couple of weeks after surgery for follow-up.

This type of surgery is usually done as an outpatient, meaning the patient will be able to go home after recovering the same day. The night before surgery, the patient may be required by her surgeon to do a bowel preparation. This varies from surgeon to surgeon, and consists of some form of clear liquid diet and laxatives to clean out the patient's colon. The patient will need assistance from family members and/or friends, as she will not be able to do much on her own for a few days and may take up to six weeks or longer to recover, depending on her doctor's instructions and what is found during surgery. It is important to follow your doctor's instructions after surgery, as this could impact your healing process.

After surgery, the patient may experience pain from surgery, nausea, and shoulder pain. The nurses can give her medications that should help with the pain and nausea. The shoulder pain is from the CO_2 gas that was used during surgery, because the gas rises in the body trying to get out, which can cause discomfort and pain.

TREATING ENDOMETRIOSIS DURING SURGERY

In this section, you will find some of the different ways surgeons choose to treat endometriosis during surgery, which include cauterization, robotic, and wide excision. Personally, I have found a wide excision laparoscopic surgery to be the most effective; I didn't have this type of surgery available before my hysterectomy, so I don't know if it would have changed my decision to have a hysterectomy. Dr. Ken Sinervo's practice website (www.centerforendo.com) provides information about different types of surgeries.

It is important to remember that surgery is not a cure for endometriosis; laparoscopic surgery is a means of treating the disease.

Cauterization Technique

Cauterization, also known as burning, coagulation, fulguration, or diathermy, is one way surgeons try to eradicate endometriosis laparoscopically. It involves burning the tissue by using a low-energy heat source to disrupt the tissue. Studies have found that burning techniques leave endometriosis behind in 80-90% of cases[1]. This is most likely because burning causes inflammation and it does not remove deep, infiltrating disease. It is important to research this type of surgery before deciding this is the method for you.

---

1   *The Endo Patient's Survival Guide: A Patient's Guide to Endometriosis & Chronic Pelvic Pain* (2015)

Samantha's Experience

As previously discussed, my first surgery was done laparoscopically by using the cauterization technique. Unfortunately, shortly after my surgery, I continued having pain, and my doctor didn't have any other treatment options for me to try. This forced me to find my second doctor, who did a second surgery and said there was no evidence that I ever had endometriosis, even though I continued to be in pain.

Robotic Technique

The robotic technique for endometriosis surgery uses a robot or computerized system to assist during laparoscopic surgery to remove the disease. This means humans are not the only ones involved in the surgery. Laparoscopic surgeries for endometriosis, as well as hysterectomies, can be performed using a robot. The da Vinci is one robotic system, in which the surgeon has control over the robot the entire time during the surgery. This method of surgery gives surgeons a 3D HD view inside the body, wristed instruments that bend and rotate far greater than the human hand, and enhanced vision, precision and control[2]. It is important to research this type of surgery before deciding this is the method for you.

Samantha's Experience

Prior to my hysterectomy, I had the option of freezing my eggs. My sister even offered to be a surrogate for me, which brought me to tears; knowing that she would do that for me meant so much. However, because of expenses, I was not able to freeze my eggs

---

2   www.davincisurgery.com/da-vinci-gynecology/endometriosis_resection.php

before my hysterectomy. At the time, I was not working and getting ready to start pharmacy school for the second time. Still, even though I wasn't able to do this, I was very thankful my sister offered to do this.

My hysterectomy was done robotically, meaning I received four incisions: one above my belly button, one where my left ovary was, one where my right ovary was, and one on my right hip. These were all glued closed afterwards, instead of being stitched or stapled. My bladder did not have to be tacked, thankfully, as I had never been pregnant; tacking a bladder after delivering a baby is sometimes necessary to prevent urinary incontinence and bladder prolapse (depending on how the baby is delivered).

The doctor determined that my right ovary and uterus were both too far gone to save, but at first my left ovary looked to be salvageable. However, after moving my left ovary he found that the back was covered in endometriosis, meaning that both ovaries would need to be removed, regardless of personal preference. Afterwards, he informed me that it would have been very hard to get pregnant with how much endometriosis there was on my ovaries and uterus. Even just removing the endometriosis off of those organs wouldn't have been sufficient; I am sure they would have still been damaged beyond the ability to safely carry a child to term. He also said that I did not have any visible endometriosis anywhere but on those three organs.

During my hysterectomy, my cervix was also removed. While this effectively meant that I did not have any woman parts left, I thought it was for the best; I did not want to have to worry about getting cervical cancer.

All that being said, you know your body better than anyone. Do not stop until you get the answers you want. Just because I had a hysterectomy does not mean you will need one.

HYSTERECTOMIES

A hysterectomy is a surgical operation in which a surgeon removes a patient's uterus, one or both ovaries, and possibly her cervix. The patient can choose if she wants to keep one of her ovaries to make sure her body can still naturally produce some level of estrogen. Once a hysterectomy is performed, the patient will not be able to have children. A hysterectomy will not guarantee a patient will no longer suffer with endometriosis, as that would require the surgeon to also remove all disease during the hysterectomy. Otherwise, the implants that are left behind will continue to grow; endometriosis makes its own estrogen, which is what the disease needs to survive. If all of the disease is removed, the patient *could* be pain free, but the decision should not be made lightly, as she will no longer be able to have children and will put herself at the beginning of menopause, no matter how old she is.

During my hysterectomy, the surgeon didn't remove all of the disease, which is why I had to have a fifth surgery. I didn't know this until I started having pain again about six months after my hysterectomy. Before my hysterectomy, I decided I wanted both of my ovaries removed because they both were very painful; we discussed keeping one of my ovaries, which would then act as two ovaries and produce the needed hormones for my body. However, he also said that this was up to me, and that I could let him know my decision at my pre-op appointment. He warned me, however, that even if I decided I wanted to keep my left ovary, if after opening me up he felt it was not salvageable, he would go ahead and remove it, so that I would not have to have surgery again. He also said that with my uterus removed, I would not need as high a dose of progesterone as I was taking.

I want to highlight here the relief that I experienced having found a physician who would take me seriously and who believed in doing what was necessary to eliminate my pain. While it can be difficult (it sure was for me), it *is* worth it to keep looking until you find a doctor who is willing to act as a real partner in your care. By the end of my first visit, I no longer cared how far I had to drive to go see him. A doctor who will listen to what you want is very valuable.

Samantha's Experience

When I first made the decision to have a hysterectomy, I was heartbroken. I felt empty; like I was somehow not good enough to be allowed the ability to get pregnant and have a child. I knew that I would never get to experience being pregnant or childbirth, but I also knew that my body would not be able to handle the rigors of pregnancy or birth; it could barely handle the pain it was in now. I had to be willing to give myself a chance at having a life.

Once I decided to have a hysterectomy, there was no talking me out of it; I was done with the pain and wanted it over as soon as possible. My body seemed to be in agreement; over the following two months, I had six periods, which is ridiculous.

It's possible that had I received proper treatment for my endometriosis from the start, I would never have reached the point of needing a hysterectomy. All

I knew at the time was that I could not bear the pain any longer; after doing any physical activity, my entire body would hurt the next day.

However, before my doctor would schedule me for the procedure, she requested that I speak to a counselor first. I remember feeling so shocked when she told me that; it made me feel as though I were back to square one, with a doctor who didn't believe the things I was telling her about my own body.

Once off the phone, I started crying, because that is what I do when I get angry. It felt like I cried for at least two hours; I was just so mad and upset that I had come this far and, just like that, I was no longer having a hysterectomy like I thought I would be; the office originally had me scheduled for a presacral neurectomy, even though I talked with her about a hysterectomy at my last appointment. Not to mention, the doctor instructed me to see the counselor at least twice, and then have the counselor write a letter saying that I understood what I was giving up by having the procedure. This made me feel like the doctor thought I was a complete idiot for making this decision. Needless to say, I did not take this news very well; I was absolutely fed up with my difficulties in finding even a single sympathetic doctor.

All of this goes to show just how little control patients have over their own healthcare. It's bad enough that women with endometriosis have seemingly no control over their body; having no control over their own treatment is almost too much to accept. Judging from my doctor's actions, it was apparently okay if my uterus fell out (as she wanted me to have a procedure done that could lead to uterine prolapse), but not okay that I wanted my uterus removed. I felt as though she also needed to cover herself for the mistakes her and her office previously made regarding scheduling.

Let me also say that I do not have anything against counselors; I think it is a good idea for people to seek counseling for help with their feelings. What I *do* have a problem with is being forced by my gynecologist to go to counseling because of my age, gender, and choice of operation. From my perspective, it is my life and my choice; I am the one living in agonizing pain every day, not them.

Because of all this, I had to wait longer to have the operation done, which meant I had to continue to put my life on hold, all while in agonizing pain. Needless to say, after this situation (which had also involved some difficulties with acquiring proper insurance), I lost what little faith I had in our current healthcare system.

WIDE EXCISION TECHNIQUE

Wide excision surgery is usually performed by endometriosis specialists. These are doctors whose only focus is treating endometriosis patients, which is what patients need—they are far more knowledgeable on all things related to the disease than standard doctors. They are usually surgeons focused on eradicating the disease by surgery. (Dr. Sinervo, who wrote the foreword for this book, is one of these surgeons.)

During excision, either mechanical energy (scissors) or a high-energy heat source (such as laser and electro surgery) is used to cut out the diseased tissue, leaving only healthy tissue behind[3]. Ablative vaporization can be used if there is a major concern that a woman's fertility will be compromised or there is a higher risk of complications during surgery.

It can be difficult to find an endometriosis specialist who uses wide excision during laparoscopic surgery to treat endometriosis, because not many surgeons use this practice. It is important to research this type of surgery before deciding this is the method for you.

Samantha's Experience

My fifth and sixth surgeries were both performed by surgeons using wide excision surgery if and when endometriosis was found. The fifth surgeon was an endometriosis specialist, and my sixth surgeon was a gynecologist. I did not have any endometriosis found during my sixth surgery, which I believe is because I had previously had wide excision surgery performed. I had some scar tissue and had to have my gallbladder removed.

Before I could have my fifth surgery, I had to take Estrace (an estrogen oral tablet) to actually *feed* my endometriosis. The idea was to make sure that the disease had grown large enough to be visible to the specialist. Each day that I took Estrace, my pain continued to worsen.

I felt stupid. I'd truly believed I had beat endometriosis by having a hysterectomy. I would look in the mirror and not recognize myself because of all the pain and hurt that I'd come through and that awaited me in the future. I could not work because of the pain, so I had to rely on my parents for financial help

---

3   *The Endo Patient's Survival Guide: A Patient's Guide to Endometriosis & Chronic Pelvic Pain* (2015)

until I started school online in a few months. That hurt in its own way; I'd always wanted to be independent, but because of my endometriosis, that didn't seem possible.

There were days where I felt I was stuck going around in circles, over and over again. I could not stand it. I was tired of not being able to enjoy life; I felt like my life was passing me by.

It was at this point that I knew I needed to make some major decisions. Was I going to continue seeing the doctors available in my area? Was I going to have a fifth surgery with a specialist? Was I going to go back to pharmacy school after my medical leave of absence? Should I change my major to something more practical for my body to handle? All these decisions to make, none of which I would have had to face were it not for my endometriosis.

In the end, I decided to go with my gut feeling and have the surgery with the endometriosis specialist. When I woke up after the surgery, I remember being in pain, but it was a different type of pain than I was used to. I was hooked up to a Dilaudid pump that I could use every ten minutes for pain if I needed to. I was not nauseous at all, which could be because a nurse put a scopolamine patch behind my ear before my surgery. I was moved from the recovery room to a private room, where I would stay overnight. While I was in the hospital, I was given Lyrica, since the doctor cut nerves that were once connected to my uterus. I also continued taking Estrace and was given a prescription for Percocet for after my discharge.

The doctor told me he excised all the endometriosis he saw. He also looked at my bladder and saw that it was smaller than normal, and diagnosed me with mild interstitial cystitis and retroperitoneal fibrosis. Interstitial cystitis is inflammation of the bladder, which can be caused by certain foods or drinks. Retroperitoneal fibrosis is a hardening around the ureters, the tubes that carry urine from the kidneys to the bladder. Both of these conditions are rare, and available information can be scarce. I was told not to worry about doing anything for these conditions, and that the doctor had stretched my bladder some to try to make it bigger. The surgery required three incisions: one at my belly button and one at each hip.

CONTINUING CARE AFTER SURGERY

I was so ready to be on hormones after my fifth surgery, but first I had to do a saliva test and wait for the results to come back. I was having terrible headaches and mood swings since I was not taking any hormones at this time. I had to collect saliva when I woke up, at noon, before dinner, and before I went to sleep.

When the results came in, my estrogen levels were in range, as were my testosterone and DHEA levels. My cortisol levels were checked at the four different times of the day I collected, and found that my morning and evening cortisol levels were high, which meant my body was stressed at those times. My cortisol levels at lunch time and before I went to bed were in range. My progesterone levels were high, but we were unsure why.

Once my doctor signed off on the recommendations, I had to make an appointment to meet with the pharmacist to get my compounded bio-identical hormones. All I knew was that I did not want to be on any estrogen; I did not want to take any chances with any endometriosis coming back! I was put on 20mg of progesterone cream at night to see if this would help my headaches. I was also put on 150mg of progesterone capsules to help me go to sleep. I was given Relora Plex to take in the morning and at lunch time to decrease my body's stress. I took 5000 IU of Vitamin D to take in the morning, and calcium to help my bones.

I saw an immediate difference in my sleep. I was able to go to sleep faster, though I was still waking up tired. However, I started feeling really nauseous after a few days of being on the hormones. I decided to stop them to see if my nausea would decrease, and after a couple of days without them, I felt a lot better. This in turn made me question whether I needed to be on all the hormones I was taking.

Follow-Up Surgeries
In 2016, I was required to have an additional sixth surgery to address some of the complications I'd experienced after my previous procedure. During surgery, my surgeons found that my gallbladder was stuck to my bowels and that my bile duct was clogged. As a result, they removed my gallbladder and, since their position had been shifted, my bowels were moved back to where they were supposed to be.

My gynecologist removed scar tissue/adhesions and found two places that needed to be biopsied. She thought they were ovarian tissue, but wanted to be sure. I was surprised to hear this; I knew the only way there could be any ovarian tissue found is if the gynecologist did not remove all of the tissue when both of my ovaries were removed, something called **ovarian remnant syndrome**, which should have been caught by my fifth surgeon. When the results came back, the gynecologist saw no evidence of any endometriosis during the surgery.

I woke up in recovery and was not in pain, but I was very nauseous. The nurses loaded me up on nausea medication and sent me home with prescriptions for Zofran (for nausea) and

Percocet (for pain). I also needed to take a stool softener, as per usual following one of my surgeries. I had four incisions, though three of them were the same incisions used for my hysterectomy (the other was just below my chest, where they removed my gallbladder.)

My post-op appointments were scheduled two weeks after my surgery. At each appointment, I made sure to ask each doctor for my surgery reports. I prayed this would be my last surgery *ever*. I am very thankful that both my gynecologist and general surgeon listened to me and did what they needed to help me feel better. I feel like they are among the few doctors I did not have to argue with or defend myself against.

My first post-op appointment was with the general surgeon who removed my gallbladder. I was so excited to tell him how much better I felt after the surgery, and asked when I could start taking baths. He was happy to hear I was feeling better, said my incisions looked great and that I could take a bath, though I still could not lift anything over twenty pounds for four more weeks. He said that my gallbladder had been inflamed and was lined with the substance that creates gallstones, so I made the right decision to have it removed. After this appointment, I cried on the way home. I was so happy to be feeling better, even though I was still sore.

My gynecologist's post-op appointment was the next day. I made a list of questions to ask her, including my hot flashes, the tissue she'd found, and my bowels. At the appointment, my iron was checked and was found to be normal. The biopsy turned out to be thick scar tissue, not ovarian tissue, but she'd wanted to make sure. The doctor did a pelvic exam and checked my incisions and said everything looked good. I asked her about taking estrogen and she said that I should still consider it, and listed its benefits. However, she added that estrogen can cause gallbladder issues, which is probably why I started having pain where my gallbladder was when I started estrogen.

RECOVERY AFTER SURGERY

Recovery after having surgery can be difficult, depending on how extensive and thorough the surgery is. Your doctor will tell you how long your recovery could take and how much time you may need to take off from work. Watching movies is a good way to relax after surgery. It is important to not overdo it.

A heating pad and comfortable clothes are essential; it is also important to get up and walk around a little bit each day to build up your stamina and prevent blood clots. Pain medicine usually makes people rest, which is a good thing because this will allow your body to heal. It is important to take your medicine as your doctor prescribes it. You won't be able to take a bath or a shower for a few days because of your incisions. If possible, have someone at home with you to help you. You may not have much of an appetite the day after surgery, but it is important to stay hydrated.

Samantha's Experience

Waking up after my hysterectomy, I already felt better, as far as my pain was concerned. My family and friends stayed in touch with me to see how I was doing and sent me things, which I am very thankful for.

The first night after the surgery was somewhat terrible. I could not go to the bathroom by myself, even though my bladder was full. My mother, who stayed the night with me, would turn on the shower, hoping the sound of water would help, but no such luck. Finally, a nurse catheterized me, and I peed 800 ml! After that, my bladder needed to rest, so I ended up having to be catheterized for the entire night. It was removed the next morning, and by then I was able to pee by myself. We went home the next day.

During my recovery after my hysterectomy, I was

put on a large amount of morphine so that when I woke up I would not be in pain. I was also given Dilaudid with Benadryl, because the pain medicine made me itch, as well as a stool softener, ibuprofen, and Zofran (for my nausea). When I was sent home, I was given prescriptions to continue these medications.

I do not remember much from the two-hour ride home form the hospital, at least in part because of the pain medication I was taking. Once home, I tried not to take Dilaudid unless I had to; I did not like the way it made me feel or that I had to take it with Benadryl to prevent itchiness.

Thankfully, my post-surgery recovery was largely uneventful. The iodine put on my incisions to help clean them was hard to get off my skin; I lost my voice after surgery because I'd had to be intubated when I was put under anesthesia; my incisions itched terribly after about a week, but I wasn't allowed to scratch them; and I needed to take laxatives on occasion (in addition to stool softeners) to have bowel movements.

But I already felt better. My doctor said that I looked better now than I did at my first appointment. I know that I made the right decision. Now it is just a question of finding the right mix of hormones to live as normal a life as I can.

Constipation

Three weeks after my surgery, I had an appointment with my doctor, who said everything looked fine. By this point, I was having regular bowel movements, so I didn't have any immediate concerns. However, four weeks after my surgery I was very constipated, despite taking a stool softener and Miralax.

At first, I was not worried; I have never been one to have a bowel movement every day. However, I was also taking 400mg of magnesium as part of my hormone therapy, which is supposed to keep you regular. I suspect I owed my constipation to the amount of Zofran I was taking to keep from vomiting.

I think the reason I felt so nauseous during that time is because my hormones were all out of whack. Once I started taking hormone medication, my nausea almost immediately subsided.

For reference, I was taking:

- Biest, 1mg cream (a form of estrogen)

- Testosterone, 1.5mg cream

- DHEA, 6mg cream

- Progesterone, 150mg capsule

- Progesterone, 50mg cream

- Magnesium, 400mg

- Phosphatidyl Serine, 150mg capsule

To resolve my constipation, I had to use an enema, which was very painful; this, on top of the pain I was already in from having had surgery, meant I was very uncomfortable. It did not seem to matter what position I was in; no matter how I sat, I had shooting pains up my rectum. I knew what I had to do, of course; but I so desperately did not want to have to give myself an enema that I kept putting it off. Performing an enema is hard enough on its own; when you have just had surgery, it's twice as painful and awkward. I had to do one before my colonoscopy almost four years prior, but I had forgotten how excruciating it can be.

It is possible to have scar tissue or adhesions appear after surgery, which can be painful. Ask your doctor about your chances of developing scar tissue after surgery, and research it as well. It is important to research the risks of having surgery, as well as talking to your doctor about them. I can't stress enough how important it is to be your own health advocate and to do your own research before agreeing to any treatment option.

DILATION AND CURETTAGE (D&C)

Dilation and curettage (or D&C) is a surgical procedure in which the cervix is opened (dilated) and a thin instrument inserted to remove tissue from the inside of the uterus (curettage). This procedure is used to treat conditions that affect the uterus, such as abnormal bleeding, and may be recommended to someone complaining of endometriosis symptoms to help rule out alternate diagnoses. Some women with endometriosis have also had this operation done to make sure there is not anything in the uterus that should not be.

PRESACRAL NEURECTOMY/NERVE ABLATION

A presacral neurectomy can be done if patients still have pain after trying surgery and other treatment options for their endometriosis, and for those who may suffer with adenomyosis, which will be discussed later. This type of procedure involves cutting the nerves connected to the uterus to stop their signaling, usually through laparoscopic incisions. This allows these nerves to stop signaling to the patient's brain that there is uterus pain. A helpful resource is centerforendo.com/presacral-neurectomy/.

> ### Samantha's Experience
> Personally, I do not have any experience with this. One of my doctors recommended that I have this done before my hysterectomy, but I didn't want to take the risk. However, it can be helpful for patients. As always, it is important to research this type of surgery before deciding this is the method for you.

4

Non-Surgical Treatment Options

OVER THE course of my battle with endometriosis, I have been through so many different treatments that I'm surprised my body has not completely shut down. In my opinion, many of the medical treatments widely available for endometriosis are not ideal for our bodies. Hopefully, my knowledge of and experience with these treatment options will help you to make an informed decision about what is best for your body. Remember: nobody knows how your body feels better than you do. Always keep that in mind.

I also want to empower you to do your own research on your best treatment options. Do not make your decision using only the information I have provided, or the information that your doctor tells you. Become an active participant in your own care! Likewise, do not be afraid to tell your doctor you want to research a recommended treatment before you try it. If anything, they should encourage you to do your own research so that you know everything there is to know about endometriosis and the treatments that could possibly alleviate your pain.

Finally, remember that everybody is different; there is no one set treatment that will help every patient. It is important to bear this in mind as you research treatment results.

LUPRON

Lupron is an injection medication that can be used to treat endometriosis and uterine fibroids (as well as prostate cancer, which is why it is so controversial). For treatment of endometriosis, the medication works by shutting down the ovaries so that women do not have a period for a certain amount of time. This stops the ovaries from producing estrogen, which stops the growth of endometriosis and sends the woman into medically-induced menopause. The medication is also thought to decrease and possibly even eliminate endometriosis implants.

This is the current working theory of Lupron usage in the treatment of endometriosis. There are different doses and frequencies that can be given at the doctor's office, depending on what the doctor is trying to accomplish. Additionally, once the medication has left the body, all normal functions should resume as they were before the medication was administered.

Doctors have claimed that Lupron does not affect a woman's ability to become pregnant and have children. However, there are serious side effects that can occur because of this medication. These side effects include osteoporosis or bone weakness, cavities, depression, and hot flashes, as well as others. Before agreeing to take this medication, be sure to do your own research to determine if it is the best fit for your body.

Samantha's Experience

I have tried many treatments in my attempts to alleviate my pelvic pain. One that I am not particularly proud of is the Lupron Depot injection. As a guideline, a woman is only allowed to have a total of twelve injections of Lupron during her lifetime. I view this as a big red flag; if a treatment was truly good for you, there would not be a limit on how many injections you could have. Yet some women may feel that this is the only option they have left, other than a full hysterectomy, which is how I felt when I tried Lupron.

I had two different rounds of Lupron injections in the hopes that I would be pain-free. The first time, after two injections which lasted for three months apiece, I *did* feel a little better. In fact, I found more relief from the Lupron than anything else I'd tried up to that point. However, during my second treatment in 2013, I found I suffered *more* pain after the first injection. I was scheduled to get a second injection three months later, but decided against it. Doctors do not always clearly explain the horrible side effects that can occur as a result of this shot. After all, putting a young woman who wants to eventually have kids through menopause is not ideal.

Symptoms that women will most likely experience while on the shot (as well as during the withdrawal period) are hot flashes, night sweats, fatigue, and pain. Because Lupron shuts down a woman's ovaries, she will not have a period during this time, and the lining of her uterus will be very thin. (The doctor that injected my final Lupron shot actually told me my uterus resembled a 70-year-old woman's. Needless to say, I did not go back for my second shot—or back to that doctor.)

Many patients are told, as I was, that Lupron will kill their endometriosis, and that while this will cause more pain in the short term, the pain should get better once the disease is gone. This was not my experience; after my second treatment, the pain was so bad I could hardly stand up and go to work. Even

getting out of bed every day was sometimes very difficult. My doctor even recommended surgery, which
would have been my fourth procedure in three years.
Thankfully, I ended up not going the surgical route
at that time.

PREMARIN/PREMPRO

These prescription medications are usually given to women
who are going through menopause to help with their hot
flashes and other symptoms. Women who have endometriosis
and have been administered Lupron may be offered this as a
treatment for their hot flashes. Premarin comes in a tablet or
cream, while Prempro is a tablet. These medications are com-
posed of conjugated estrogen in the form of urine from pregnant horses. The estrogen that a woman's body produces is not
in the same form as Premarin or Prempro, which may cause
side effects. Before agreeing to try either one of these medications, be sure to do your own research to determine if it is the
best fit for your body.

Samantha's Experience

When I went to the Mayo Clinic, the doctor I saw
there wanted me to take Prempro, as I was still technically in menopause from a Lupron shot. However,
I did not take him up on this offer; while Premarin
and Prempro *do* have small amounts of estrogen, because the drugs are manufactured from horse urine,
it can be harmful. These two medications are prescribed to many women because doctors receive
special reimbursement for each prescription they
write.

DEPO PROVERA

Depo Provera is a form of birth control given as a progestin injection, which lasts for three months each time it is given. This can be beneficial for women who have a hard time remembering to take a pill every day and are not interested in a birth control patch. Side effects include weight gain, hair loss, depression, and nausea, as well as symptoms from other forms of birth control.

It can be helpful for endometriosis patients because it prevents ovulation, since the shot is a continuous form of birth control every three months. Before agreeing to try this prescription medication, be sure to do your own research to determine if it is the best fit for your body.

> *Samantha's Experience*
> Depo Provera did nothing to help my pain, though it *did* cause me to shed a lot of hair. What's more, with both Lupron and Depo Provera, I experienced burning at the injection site and could not sit on my hip for a couple of days. This can be especially aggravating if, like me, you have to sit in class or at work for hours at a time.

BIRTH CONTROL PILLS

Containing both estrogen and progesterone, birth control bills are designed to prevent pregnancy and are often prescribed to help regulate periods. The hope is that by shutting down the ovaries, you disable the endometriosis and inhibit its ability to grow any further.

Birth controls come in different dosages, which can be helpful for patients with endometriosis to determine the lowest dose of estrogen they can tolerate and still receive the benefits.

Remember, estrogen *feeds* endometriosis. Some endometriosis patients may benefit if their birth control is continuous, which means the last row of pills would be skipped and the patient would start the next pack of birth control pills.

Side effects include blood clots, nausea, weight gain, depression, headaches, chest pain, and swelling. The hormones in birth controls are not similar to what our bodies naturally make, so before agreeing to try any of these prescription medications, be sure to do your own research to determine if it is the best fit for your body.

Samantha's Experience

My doctor prescribed me the birth control pill Necon, during the use of which I still managed to have a period even though I was only taking the active pills and skipping the last week of pills of each pack. I also found that birth control made my acne worse. Even though I tried several different birth controls, none of them decreased my pain.

OTHER PILLS USED TO TREAT PAIN

There are a seemingly endless variety of both prescription and over-the-counter pills that claim to treat almost any kind of pain.

Nonsteroidal Anti-inflammatory Drugs (NSAIDs): These are common pain medications that are prescribed to help alleviate endometriosis pain. Examples of these include ibuprofen (Motrin, Advil), naproxen (Aleve), meloxicam (Mobic) and Celebrex. They work by reducing inflammation in the body, which could be caused by endometriosis. Celebrex is usually prescribed for arthritis, but has been tried for endometriosis pain, as well.

Opioids: Opioids are another type of medication that may help alleviate pain for a little while. These include tramadol (Ultram), hydrocodone (Vicodin, Norco), oxycodone (Percocet), fentanyl (Duragesic) patches, hydromorphone (Dilaudid), and morphine (Roxanol). These pain medications work in endometriosis patients by minimizing pain signals to different parts of the body and reduce the pain.

Antidepressants: Cymbalta and Elavil, two medications usually used to treat depression, can also be used to treat chronic pain.

However, even the most effective pain pills do not fix the problem. Rather, they cover up the problem—kind of like a Band-Aid. They may make you feel better for a little while, but that will not last long-term. This is why people become addicted to painkillers; their doctors prescribe them some type of pain medication, which *seems* to make the pain go away, so they continue to take them until they cannot function without them. Many doctors may also refuse to prescribe pain killers to endometriosis patients, for fear that the medication is being abused. In reality, it is the severity and consistency of pain that these patients suffer that give off the appearance of pain killer addiction or abuse.

Before agreeing to try any of these prescription medications, be sure to do your own research to determine if it is the best fit for your body.

Samantha's Experience

Medications that I have personally used to try to minimize pain include:

- Ibuprofen (Motrin)
- Naproxyn (Aleve)
- Tylenol with Codeine
- Ponstel
- Percocet
- Tramadol
- Hydrocodone
- Celebrex
- Meloxicam
- Dilaudid
- Lidocaine Patches
- Cyclobenazeprine (Flexeril) (technically a muscle relaxer)

Of these, Tylenol with Codeine, Dilaudid, and Percocet are the only three pain pills that have come close to taking the edge off, as far as my endometriosis pain is concerned. One of my doctors prescribed me NSAIDS and antidepressants to see if they would help with my endometriosis pain, but after taking them for a few months, I saw no improvement and discontinued the treatment. I did not like the way opioids made me feel, so I only took them when I couldn't bear the pain any longer.

5

Alternative Medicine

BIO-IDENTICAL HORMONE THERAPY

Our bodies make hormones that help regulate the body's functions. All of the hormones in our bodies play a collective role in how we feel every day. If one hormone is out of whack, that can cause other hormones to have problems, which can lead to us feeling bad.

When speaking about endometriosis, the two main hormones to consider are the body's main sex hormones. Sex hormones are the same in both women and men; they're just found in different amounts. In women, progesterone and estrogen are the two main sex hormones. Many women become estrogen dominant, which means that there is too much estrogen in the body. This is what happens to those of us who suffer with endometriosis. Too much estrogen has also been known to cause cancer. Progesterone, by contrast, is the "natural healer" hormone. If a body contains more progesterone than estrogen, that's ideal; progesterone is known to decrease night sweats, hot flashes, fatigue, headaches, and other symptoms caused by too much estrogen.

To address the sorts of hormone imbalances found with endometriosis, one option is through the use of bio-identical hormone treatment. Bio-identical hormones, as differentiated from "natural hormones," means the hormones are in some way artificial, or man-made (natural hormones are still produced, but come from natural sources such as plants or animal urine). The advantage of bio-identical hormones is that they're much closer to what your body makes itself, and is therefore much easier for your body to recognize and use as it needs to.

Unfortunately, many doctors do not understand the proper use of bio-identical hormones, which is why so many women suffer from estrogen dominance. In truth, it is much easier to adjust a dosage of a bio-identical hormone than a pharmaceutical form of a hormone such as Premarin, which can be prescribed as an oral tablet or vaginal cream.

Samantha's Experience

When I first started using progesterone cream, I needed to have my dosage tweaked quite a few times before finding one that worked. When I first started using it, I was still having headaches after using it one time each day. My doctor then wanted me to halve the prescribed dose and apply that amount twice daily, which helped minimize the headaches.

You must make sure to rub all bio-identical hormone creams in well, because if you do not, they can transfer to another person or clothing. It can be very aggravating, having to rub cream on your arm, ovaries, or forehead (depending on where your doctor tells you to use it) once or twice a day. It is very annoying when you are on vacation, like at the beach or lake, and have to stop what you are doing and make sure it dries before you get in the water or lay out in the sun, but it is worth it.

Because my dose of progesterone needed to be so high, the cream was thick, which makes it harder for it to absorb quickly into the skin and get where it needs to go. But even though it can be a hassle, I knew if I did not use it like I was supposed to, I would feel the pain later (literally).

If you are interested in talking to your doctor about hormones or other treatment options, I highly recommend reading *The Miracle of Bio-identical Hormones,* by renowned medical specialist Dr. Michael Platt, and *Stop Endometriosis and Pelvic Pain: What Every Woman & Her Doctor Need to Know,* by well-known endometriosis specialist Dr. Andrew Cook, who practices in California. More books on endometriosis are provided in the Resources and Relevant Research section at the end of this book.

Hormone Testing for Using Bio-identical Hormones

Hormone levels can be tested using three methods: blood, urine, and saliva testing. In my experience, testing hormones via saliva is the best route, because the test results will show how much of the hormone is free, or waiting to be used, which in turn shows how much is available to bind at the body's receptor sites. Urine testing, which is often expensive and much more time-consuming, shows what hormones are currently being metabolized. Finally, blood testing results show the number of hormones that are already bound at the receptor sites. Women with endometriosis will usually present with very low progesterone levels and abnormally high levels of estrogen, regardless of which test is performed.

Samantha's Experience

I have had many blood tests done by different doctors and was told that everything was normal, except that my Vitamin D levels were too low. This has been found to be low in women who suffer from endometriosis. I was left to wonder how everything could be normal if I was in so much agonizing pain. It wasn't until I received a saliva test through the pharmacy I worked for that I got a real picture of my hormone levels: my progesterone was so low, it is a wonder I was not showing more symptoms. My estrogen was also higher than it should be, which could create more problems down the road, including cancer. My testosterone was also high, which is why I have had problems with acne. I was put on a high enough dose of progesterone cream that I did not have a period for the first few months, which decreased the number of hot flashes and night sweats I had.

PELVIC FLOOR PHYSICAL THERAPY

As the saying goes, "Use it or lose it," and that goes double for your body. If you do not use your muscles on a regular basis, they will lose their tone and strength.

There are different techniques a physical therapist can use to help relieve pelvic pain. They will also instruct you in ways to relax your body, as well as stretches to help minimize pain and restore your range of function.

Biofeedback is one technique that is used during pelvic floor physical therapy. Using sensors positioned in the vagina, which help the physical therapist gauge how your muscles are working, how tight they are, and how often they spasm with stimulus, the physical therapist uses this information to come up with a plan to help alleviate your pain.

Connective tissue manipulation is another technique that can be used. The therapist uses lotion or lubricant to rub/massage/manipulate your abdominal, vaginal, thigh, and/or back tissue. It can be extremely painful, but you will notice the difference after each session, though how long the benefits last will differ with the individual.

As with all healing, the pain is going to get worse before it gets better. If you decide to try physical therapy for pain relief, you will most likely be in pain after several sessions. Do not get discouraged; this is common. Keep pushing through and continue to do the exercises your physical therapist gives you. There is a light at the end of the tunnel!

Doctors should allow patients to do a pelvic floor drop or squeeze before performing a gynecological exam with a speculum. This allows the patient to relax and the exam to be less painful. However, rather than take the time to do this, many doctors rush through the exam, causing the patient to tense up and jam the speculum, causing pain. Depending on the state of the patient's pelvic floor, this pain could be excruciating.

Samantha's Experience

During a visit to the Mayo Clinic in Jacksonville, FL in 2013, the doctor I was seeing noticed I had what he called "involuntary pelvic floor spasms." What this meant is that if any stimulus came in contact with my vagina, it made my pelvic floor spasm. This would happen when inserting tampons or even just from touch, such as during a pelvic exam.

I started going to a pelvic floor physical therapist once a week. I'm not going to lie—at first, I was anxious, thinking it was going to be incredibly awkward. I kept thinking, "Who in the world has to go to vagina rehab?" But as it turns out, many women and even men suffer from pelvic floor dysfunction. However, it does take time, motivation, and patience to get through the pain of the actual physical therapy.

When I first started going to physical therapy, I found that I was not breathing correctly due to the amount of pelvic pain I had. I would breathe using my chest instead of my stomach. The first exercise I was given was to practice laying down and breathing so my stomach would rise and fall. This took some time to get used to, but after some practice, I could do it without thinking about it.

I also have a list of stretches that I do every day, as well as some strengthening exercises that I do every other day as part of my physical therapy treatment. They include:

Daily Stretches
- Diaphragmatic breathing
- Pelvic floor drops
- Toilet positioning techniques
- Iliopsoas stretch
- Standing alignment
- Hamstring stretch
- Hip flexor stretch
- Double knee to chest
- Camel–Cat

Alternating Days Stretches
- Manual stretching of pelvic floor muscles
- Clam shell exercise
- Strengthening hips exercise

At the time, I was still going to physical therapy once a week. I do not recommend you do these stretches until you have consulted with your doctor and/or a physical therapist.

I am so thankful for my physical therapist. I could not believe that after just six months of physical therapy, I no longer had vaginal pain! After my last scheduled appointment in November 2013, I cried part of the way home because I was so happy; I did not know how to act with decreased pain levels! I am telling you all this because I want you to know there *is* hope for you; that you, too, can have less pain.

At-Home Remedies for Pelvic Pain

There are a variety of different things you can try to alleviate some of the endometriosis pain besides pain medication and surgery. For example, there are many naturopathic ways of dealing with the pain, which avoids the need for potentially harmful prescription medications. Ask your doctor what supplements you can add to your diet to help combat your symptoms so that you do not have to suffer the nasty side effects of pain medications. If your doctor does not agree with that approach, do research to find a doctor who will, especially if you are truly interested in exploring non-prescription medication options.

Endofemm (Pelvic Pain Solutions)

This is a heating pad that you can strap around your waist. You can either heat it in the microwave to act as a heating pad or stick it in the freezer to act as an ice pack. I have found it works really well if I heat it up for a minute in the microwave, strap it around my waist, and lay in the bed with it covered up; it seems to stay warmer this way. You can also position it so that the pad is on your back if you suffer from back pain.

Endofemm works using organic beads that heat up quickly. They are made from corn, and the cloth comes in different designs made from cotton fleece. With this heating pad, you will not have to worry about finding an outlet near you to plug it in or remembering to turn it off. I consider it to be the best heating pad for those who suffer with pelvic or back pain. Pelvic Pain Solutions also has ice packs that you can straddle, comfortable clothing, seat cushions, and many more helpful items for those that suffer from any type of pelvic pain.

Endovan (Komodo Nutraceuticals)

Endovan is a natural supplement which, prior to my research for this book, I had never heard of. It contains safe, all-natural ingredients including vitamin B6, Nattokinase NSP-2, *vibumum opulus* (cramp bark), Lycopene, and *vitex agnus-castus* (chasteberry). The supplement is also gluten- and dairy-free, which caught my attention; it can be hard to find supplements that do not contain gluten or dairy ingredients.

After three days of taking Endovan, I did not feel as bloated or have as much cramping. I had more energy, and my ovaries were not as sore. After a few weeks of taking the supplement, my ovary pain was minimal, less than it had been in a long time. However, when it was time for my period, I found I was still in quite a lot of pain. Hopefully, the pain will ease off after taking the supplement for a few months.

Since starting Endovan, I have gone down one pant size and have lost almost five pounds in my stomach. My stomach does not look as bloated or swollen as before. I am not saying everyone will have these results, but I think it is worth looking into and possibly trying. It is somewhat expensive—$50 for a bottle of 60 capsules, which lasts for a month—so I recommend talking to your doctor about it to make sure it's right for you.

Massages

You may find that a therapeutic massage helps with your pain. These can also help relieve pressure points and stress. Usually, a professional therapeutic massage will be an hour long, during which time, the massage therapist will do everything to make sure you are relaxed.

Of course, during the massage itself, you may not feel relief if you have pain present in a certain area. However, after the massage, the pain should be relieved (depending on how much pain you were in before and how long the massage therapist spent on that area).

Facials

Facials (together with balancing your hormones) can help tremendously with any acne or redness you may be experiencing. Your initial results may be discouraging; after my first facial, my face looked terrible—it was really red and my bumps were even more apparent. But after going every two weeks for a few months and using some acne products recommended to me by the esthetician, my acne largely cleared up without any scars. After that, I would go in for a facial once a month (until I moved in 2014). It may be a little expensive, but well worth it!

That said, just because something works for one person's acne does not mean it will work for another's. There are different reasons why people get acne; one product may help one person, while doing nothing for someone else. My advice is to find something that works for you (or find someone who knows their stuff and ask them), and stick to it!

Herbal Treatments

There are a few herbal treatment options that some women have found to be helpful in the treatment of their endometriosis symptoms. These options are intended to help decrease inflammation, which results in decreased pain—they cannot destroy endometriosis.

Dandelions/Dandelion Tea. Consuming dandelions is thought to be a helpful alternative to treating endometriosis. Dandelions are also believed to have properties that strengthen the immune system and improve liver function.

Essential Oils. Essential oils are natural oils that can be applied to different areas. Women can use these to help them relax as well as try to decrease endometriosis symptoms. Different oils have different properties, as far as how they affect the body.

Some essential oils that may help women treat their endometriosis symptoms include:

- Clary sage

- Frankincense

- Sandalwood

- Lavender

Other Herbal Treatment Options. The following is a list of some other herbal treatment options that may benefit women who suffer with endometriosis in helping treat their symptoms:

- Motherwort

- Chamomile

- Flaxseeds

- Burdock

- Milk thistle

6

How to Find the Right Doctor

My experience trying to find the right doctor has been equal parts exhausting, frustrating, and demoralizing. What I've found is that many doctors simply do not listen to their patients. They are too concerned with statistics: how many patients they can fit into one day to make the most money. It's a revolving door mentality, an assembly line approach to medicine. If they *did* care about their patients—if they felt their role was to determine the best care plan for each one—they'd likely take more than ten minutes per visit.

All the same, finding the right doctor is invaluable in your pursuit of relief from endometriosis. The majority of effective treatments, both current and experimental, will depend in part on you having a doctor who is knowledgeable, communicative, and devoted to your care. In this chapter, we'll be exploring some of the ways to locate the best fit doctor for you and your needs—and how to know when it's time to quit your current doctor.

WHAT DOCTORS DO I NEED?
There are several types of doctors that are beneficial in receiving the best healthcare possible. In my personal health journey, I've found it valuable to consult with endometriosis

specialists, family practitioners/internists, gynecologists, gastroenterologists, urologists, endocrinologists, rheumatologists, pulmonologists, and cardiologists, as well as a pelvic floor physical therapist, counselor, and pain management doctor. Quite a laundry list, but endometriosis has been found to have comorbidities, which means that there are other diseases associated with women who have endometriosis.

That's why it is important to know what each of these doctors practice to know if you might benefit from seeing any of them.

Endometriosis Specialist

When suffering with endometriosis, one of the best things a patient can do is to seek out an endometriosis specialist. This is a medical doctor who knows the ins and outs of the disease and specializes in its treatments. They usually do not use birth controls, Lupron, or other medications; instead, they use the approach of excising the disease, getting rid of the culprit in hopes of the patient living a pain-free life.

They may perform an ultrasound to determine how the uterus and ovaries look and to come up with a plan to treat the disease. Surgeons utilizing excision in their treatment plans report rates of long-term relief in 75–85 percent of their patients, while non–excisional surgery reports a 40–60 percent recurrence rate in as little as one to two years post-surgery.[4]

> *Samantha's Experience*
>
> In my experience, excision surgery has proved to be the most beneficial method for decreasing my endometriosis pain. I still have concerns about the disease coming back, because it seems like it has always reared its ugly head at the most unexpected times in

---

4   http://centerforendo.com/lapex-laparoscopic-excision-of-endometriosis/

my life. Since having excision surgery by an endometriosis specialist, I have had one surgery to remove my gallbladder and scar tissue, and have gone a year and a half without any surgery for endometriosis concerns.

Family Practioners/Internists

These doctors are beneficial for doing lab work and testing for some gastrointestinal-related issues, and can help to rule out other illnesses as well as refer patients to specialists, depending on the issue.

Samantha's Experience

The family practitioners I've seen ended up being the ones who found that I am vitamin D deficient, performed the bone scan that diagnosed me with osteoporosis, and referred me to a gastroenterologist, endocrinologist, and rheumatologist when they suspected that something else could be going on. Insurance sometimes requires these doctors to refer patients to specialists before they can cover any appointments, which can be frustrating for the patient. My doctor also likes to do blood work every six months to one year as a follow-up, which I appreciate.

Gynecologists

Gynecologists are usually the first doctors that women go to see to get birth control, oftentimes before they suspect there could be something wrong. Gynecologists specialize in womens' reproductive organs; this is where women will have their yearly pap smears, mammograms, and bone density tests done.

They may do ultrasounds, blood work, and saliva testing, as well.

> *Samantha's Experience*
>
> Even though gynecologists should specialize in women's diseases, it has been hard for me to find one that does over the course of dealing with endo-metriosis. I feel like they only want to throw birth controls or Lupron at patients in hopes of treating the disease without having to try excision surgery or refer women to an endometriosis specialist. It was difficult for me to find a gynecologist who would also treat me for PCOS, even though the illness deals with the ovaries. This was because I do not fit the appearance of a "typical" PCOS patient.

Gastroenterologists

Gastroenterologists specialize in the digestive system. This includes the esophagus, stomach, intestines, gallbladder, colon, rectum, pancreas, and liver. Diseases that they can test for include celiac disease, inflammatory bowel syndrome/disease, crohn's disease, colitis, and *h. pylori*, among others. They know how the digestive system is supposed to function and what to do to get it working properly if there is an issue.

> *Samantha's Experience*
>
> I have had two colonoscopies performed by two different gastroenterologists after being referred to check and see if my pain was due to an intestinal illness. Before my second colonoscopy, my family doctor tested me for *h. pylori* (which came back neg-

ative); I have also had a barium enema test and CT scans done with contrast, which were both normal. I am currently taking Miralax 1–3 times a day, depending on how my bowels feel from one day to the next.

Urologist

Interstitial cystitis is a common disease among women who suffer with endometriosis and can be diagnosed by a urologist or an endometriosis specialist. Urologists may perform MRIs, test for urinary tract infections, and may ask patients to keep track of how much fluid they drink versus their urine output (commonly called a bladder diary). They also perform cystoscopies and urine flow tests.

Samantha's Experience

I kept a bladder diary, had an MRI done, and had urine flow tests performed. However, my urologist told me that all of these were normal for me. I looked at my MRI results online and it said that I had free fluid in my pelvic region, which my urologist never told me about. I currently do not see a urologist; however, as with all medical practitioners, if you suspect your doctor is withholding information from you, you are better off seeking help elsewhere. A few years later, during my fifth surgery, I was diagnosed with interstitial cystitis and my bladder was expanded, but I still don't take any medications for this illness. My sister, brother, and cousins have kidney stones, which was a concern of mine, but testing showed I didn't have any kidney stones.

Endocrinologist

Endocrinologists specialize in the endocrine system, which includes hormonal imbalances and some cancers. Polycystic Ovary Syndrome (PCOS), osteoporosis, and infertility are some of the comorbidities associated with endometriosis that endocrinologists treat. They may do blood work, saliva testing, bone scans, and surgery, depending on the disease they are testing for, and will determine the best course of action if you have one of these diseases.

Samantha's Experience

In 2012, before I had my hysterectomy, I called an endocrinologist's office to see if I could make an appointment to see if I had PCOS. After I told them my medical history, for some reason they said they couldn't see me. I started seeing one in 2015, when my family doctor referred me to one after she ordered a bone scan and my T-score was in the range of osteoporosis. I discuss my experience with osteoporosis and PCOS in subsequent chapters.

Rheumatologist

Many of the other dieases that can present with or be affected by endometriosis are autoimmune in nature, which would be diagnosed and treated by a rheumatologist. An autoimmune disease is "a disorder that occurs when the body's immune system attacks and damages its own tissue"[5]. Examples of these include lupus, rheumatoid arthritis, and other illnesses associated with inflammation. Blood tests such as antinuclear antibodies (ANA) can be done to determine if a patient has an autoimmune disease and can lead to further testing depending on the result.

---

5   http://endometriosis.org/news/research/endometriosis-and-comorbidities/

Samantha's Experience

After being diagnosed with osteoporosis, I started having leg pain. I went to my family doctor and she did blood work to check to see if I had any auto-immune diseases, because she didn't think the pain was from osteoporosis. The blood work came back showing that my Antinuclear Antibody (ANA) test was positive. She referred me to a rheumatologist, though I had to wait around five months before managing to get an appointment. He completed the blood work, and all the tests came back negative. He determined that I didn't show any signs of au-toimmune diseases; despite this, my pain continued to come and go. My dad has neuropathy, which was a concern of mine, but it has been ruled out with testing, thankfully.

Pulmonologist

Asthma and allergies have been associated with endometriosis[6]. It is also rare, but possible, to have endometriosis on or around the lungs. A pulmonologist is a specialist dealing in the treatment of respiratory illnesses. Your family doctor can determine if you need to see a pulmonologist for further testing.

Samantha's Experience

This is a little aside from endometriosis, but my mom has alpha-1 antitrypsin deficiency, which affects her lungs. Her liver doesn't produce a protein that helps her lungs function. She receives weekly infusions to give her body this protein and is on continuous oxygen.

6 http://endometriosis.org/news/research/endometriosis-and-comorbidities/

I started having chest pain a few months after going to see the rheumatologist and went to see a pulmonologist. I wasn't sure if it was pain from endometriosis in my chest, heart-related, or something to do with being a carrier of alpha-1 antitrypsin deficiency. The pulmonologist ordered an EKG, which showed I had minimal mitral valve prolapse. He also conducted a lung function test, which showed my lung function was normal. I was experiencing shortness of breath when going up stairs, so he gave me an inhaler to use if I needed to and referred me to a cardiologist. Being an alpha-1 antitrypsin carrier does not relate to my endometriosis, but I wanted to include pulmonology here, as it is possible to have endometriosis that affects breathing.

Cardiologist

Endometriosis has been shown to put women at a higher risk of cardiovascular disease. Cardiologists can perform electrocardiograms (EKG), heart monitor, and stress testing for patients who have chest pain or other heart symptoms and a history of heart illness in their family. They can diagnose heart murmurs, valve malfunctions, and coronary artery disease, among other heart-related illnesses.

Samantha's Experience

The cardiologist I saw conducted a stress test, which was normal, and gave me a heart monitor to wear for a month to keep track of my chest pain and other symptoms. The monitor came with a phone that allowed me to press a button and check off any symptoms I was experiencing at that time. The results were normal, even though I experienced chest pain and an EKG showed minimal valve prolapse, so the pain was thought to be related to anxiety, which I have never been diagnosed with.

Pelvic Floor Physical Therapist

As described in Chapter 5, pelvic floor physical therapy is one alternative medicine approach that can be beneficial for those suffering with pelvic floor spasms due to endometriosis. It is important that we feel comfortable with a pelvic floor physical therapist, as these appointments can be extremely uncomfortable depending on the method being used. A gynecologist or an endometriosis specialist can refer you to a pelvic floor physical therapist in your area. They are not as common as other physical therapists, so you may have to travel depending on where you are located, but it can be worth it.

Counselor/Therapist

It is important to have a counselor, a therapist, and/or a psychiatrist to talk to about the emotions you're experiencing due to your endometriosis. It can be helpful to talk to someone who is not part of your family and gives you time for relaxation and to try different techniques that can be beneficial for relieving stress. It's also valuable to have an outlet for your feelings that won't affect anyone else. Some of these medical professionals do not prescribe medication, but can refer you to a physician who does if that is something you both agree you need. It can take up time and money depending on what your insurance will cover, but in my opinion, it is well worth it.

Samantha's Experience

I started going to a counselor about six months after being diagnosed with osteoporosis and I can feel the difference. I didn't realize how much I was keeping bottled inside, or how much my health weighs on my mind, none of which is beneficial. I have also found it helpful to read self-help books as I strive to keep a positive outlook on life every day. One book that I found helpful soon after having my hysterectomy was *The Next Happy: Let Go of the Life You Planned and Find a New Way Forward* by Tracey Cleantis. Even though I made the decision to have a hysterectomy, it was still extremely hard for me to let go of not being able to experience pregnancy and birth my own child. However, I know that I can adopt if that time comes.

Pain Management

Some patients have benefited from seeing a pain management doctor. These are doctors who will monitor patients on different pain medications to see which is the best fit. Personally, I do not have any experience with a pain management doctor.

WHEN TO QUIT YOUR DOCTOR

When being referred to specialists, it is important that you feel validated and like your concerns are taken seriously, just like when going to any other doctor. If you don't like a doctor that you have been referred to, ask your doctor who referred you for another referral, or try to see if you can find someone on your own. It is important that you have a great relationship with all of your medical providers to ensure you receive the best possible healthcare.

Many women suffer from pelvic pain, but do not know the cause or how to fix it, and so do nothing. It is time to stand up for our health instead of sitting on the sidelines! It is time that we stand up for the healthcare treatments we want instead of letting doctors decide what is best for our bodies—especially when they have no idea what we are going through.

Medical professionals need to appreciate that each patient is different. In the case of endometriosis, for example, not every patient can tolerate birth control pills, a seemingly go-to solution for many practitioners. Your hope is to find a doctor that is open-minded about potential options, with their main focus being getting the patient better.

However, a lot of money is provided to doctors by pharmaceutical companies, which in turn puts pressure on doctors to write a certain number of prescriptions for certain drugs, regardless of whether it's right for someone or puts their health at a potential risk. Also, when a drug does *not* work, your doctor should not brush off the side effects like they are nothing. This makes the patient feel like she is wrong, which results in her not wanting to mention any other side effects, which in turn puts her health at risk.

If a doctor will not listen to your symptoms or wants you to try a treatment you do not want to participate in, do not do it. They can do nothing without your consent, and there is nothing they can do (beyond refusing to treat you) if you refuse to try a treatment. If this happens, find another doctor. It might seem like a never-ending process, but keep pushing until you find a doctor you like, one that will listen to what you have to say and what you want to do.

Many women who have endometriosis choose to go to a female doctor because they believe a woman will understand more of what they're going through, as far as painful periods and cramping are concerned. But this is not always true; I have been to see male doctors who seemed to understand more of what was going on than some of the women doctors I have been to. In truth, it does not matter if the doctor is male or female. What matters is that the patient feels the doctor is respectful, has a good bedside manner, and is very knowledgeable about endometriosis, including its treatment options and the mechanics of a woman's body. It is important that patients are comfortable with their doctors so they can discuss all of their symptoms openly and honestly.

Samantha's Experience

During my search for a doctor who would take my condition seriously *and* respect my input into my care, there were many times when I felt like giving up. I was not receiving any helpful answers from doctors regarding why I was still in so much pain and what else I could try. The doctors I saw never understood that this was *my* body and I was going to do what I thought was best for it, no matter what they tried to persuade me to do. I felt like a guinea pig with all of the different treatments I tried, but I had to try something; I am not one to sit around and do nothing, especially about something as serious as my health.

BEING ACTIVE IN YOUR OWN CARE

With so many doctors out there ignorant or misinformed in regard to endometriosis and its treatment (and so few doctors willing to seriously consider a patient's input), it's important that you be ready and willing to stand up for yourself and take an active role in your care.

For example: when having your blood checked, it is important to know what to ask your doctor to check for, especially if you suspect something. Here is a list of what I typically have my doctor check and what I believe all doctors should test for:

Glucose	GGT	MCHC
Uric acid	Iron	RDW
BUN	Total Cholesterol	Platelets
Creatine	Triglycerides	Neutrophils
Sodium	HDL Cholesterol	Lymphocytes
Potassium	LDL Cholesterol	Monocytes
Chloride	Total Cholesterol/	Eosinophils
Carbon Dioxide	HDL ratio	Basophils
Calcium	TSH	Immature Granulo-
Phosphorus	Thyroxine (T4)	cytes
Protein	T3 Uptake	Free T4
Albumin	Free Thyroxine Index	Reverse T3
Globulin	White Blood Cells	Triiodothyronine
Albumin/Globulin	(WBC)	Thyroid Peroxidase
ratio	Red Blood Cells	AB (TPO AB)
Bilirubin	(RBC)	Antithyroglobulin
Alkaline phosphate	Hemoglobin	AB Siemens
LDH	Hematocrit	Free Triiodothyro-
AST	MCV	nine
ALT	MCH	

$\overline{7}$

Lifestyle Changes

E XERCISE AND diet can provide some relief from endometriosis symptoms. However, it is important to remember that lifestyle changes alone will not get rid of your disease, if they're the only element of your treatment plan. That said, it can be beneficial to establish a daily routine for yourself to help keep your pain levels at a minimum.

Exercise

Exercising can be hard to do for those of us suffering with chronic pain, whether because of endometriosis or any other type of illness. However, if you can do something for as little as an hour a day, it can be beneficial to your overall health. Being active decreases your risk of having other diseases.

Samantha's Experience

Since my sixth surgery, I have been exercising more than I have since being diagnosed with endometriosis. I was a very active child growing up, but once I started having my period, it became harder for me to be active.

I completely relate to not feeling well enough to

get out of bed, let alone exercise. However, since I've
started exercising, I can feel a difference in my body
and stamina. Even though I am tired after working
out, I still have more energy overall. I have also attended yoga classes that have been very relaxing for
me and find them not to be as strenuous as other
workouts.

DIET

Diet can play a big role in pain levels and overall health. There
are foods that are thought to be triggers for endometriosis
flares and other related illnesses, including red meats, processed
foods, sugar, soy, dairy, caffeine, and alcohol. All of these foods
have chemicals that are hard for our bodies to process and can
cause inflammation. It is important to drink as much water as
possible because it will help flush out toxins. Organic foods are
another, much healthier alternative to the trigger foods, as they
can come from local sources and have little, if any, pesticides.

Gluten-Free/Dairy-Free Diet

It is hard to imagine life without bread. Yet more and more
people are discovering that their bodies are intolerant of gluten. Gluten products include anything which contains wheat,
barley, or rye. Many people are unable to digest these food ingredients, which causes inflammation and pain. However, that
doesn't mean you need to go hungry or have a strict and lim-
iting diet. Look for gluten-free breads that you can either buy
or cook yourself to replace your white or wheat breads. There
are also gluten-free pastas available to replace standard maca-
roni and cheese and other pastas, and even gluten-free pizza
crusts you can buy or prepare. There are gluten-free desserts
like cookies, cakes, and brownies, or you could limit yourself to
fruits and vegetables. (A great resource on how to maintain a

gluten-free diet is Elisabeth Hasselbeck's book *The G-Free Diet: A Gluten-Free Survival Guide*, which describes her struggles to find a diagnosis for her pelvic pain as well as finding the foods that are right for her body. She also goes through what foods are good, which are bad, and how you can live gluten-free.)

Dairy is another pain trigger for many people. Thankfully, there are a wide variety of lactose-free products, including milks, cheeses, ice cream, yogurt, and butters. My favorite brand of dairy-free gluten-free ice cream, milk, and yogurt is So Delicious. It tastes just as good, if not better, than regular ice cream, and the company makes their products using coconut milk. Almond or coconut milk is a milk alternative that tastes very good *and* is better for you than dairy milk. Vegan butter is a good replacement for dairy butter; I also use it to wipe down pans before I cook with them so food does not stick. There is also coconut oil, which you can cook with and use in certain recipes.

Truly healthy food can be somewhat of a challenge to find, but once you find a store you like, you can just shop there instead of other grocery stores. Gluten-free food can be found at health food stores or organic food stores such as Trader Joe's, Whole Foods, or Fresh Market. There are also some restaurants that have gluten-free and dairy-free menus in addition to other food allergy menus that you can order from. If you are intolerant to gluten, dairy, or any other food product, you will have to be very careful when it comes to cross-contamination. Cross-contamination means that if something that contains gluten comes into contact with gluten-free food, the gluten-free food has been contaminated and should not be consumed by someone who cannot eat gluten. The same is true for dairy and dairy-free food. You may find you need to ask a bunch of questions to make sure the cooks are cautious when preparing your meal, and while that may seem like a hassle now, it will be well worth it if it keeps you safe and pain-free.

Samantha's Experience

For a couple of months before I went gluten-free, I kept a journal of what medicines I took, what I ate, my symptoms, and the times of each. I noticed I felt groggy after I ate and continued to feel that way for the rest of the day. I also had frequent headaches after eating. I know now one of the culprits was gluten. I tried taking a Glutenease supplement, which is supposed to help process gluten-containing foods; however, I did not see any difference in my pain.

Keeping a health journal in this way can be an invaluable aid, both to you and to your doctors, as you try to track down exactly what triggers your symptoms.

Organic Foods

In addition to knowing what foodstuffs to avoid, it is also important to know which foods to look for. Do not be afraid to try new and better foods! You owe it to yourself to make your body feel better. The saying "you are what you eat" is very true. For example, while organic foods can be somewhat pricey, they are always better for you. There are many gluten-free and dairy-free options, as well as soy-free options (soy is an unhealthy additive used to make ingredients stick together).

Let me stress one thing: changing your diet is *not* a cure for endometriosis. It *has* been known to help some women's pain levels decrease, but that does not mean their disease is gone; it means their inflammation has been decreased, leading to some relief. There is no known cure for endometriosis. In short, a change in diet is a possible treatment for women with endometriosis that may decrease pain, but it will not decrease the amount of endometriosis or scar tissue in the body.

STRESS

Stressing and worrying about everything is no way to live; it will catch up with you sooner or later, causing your body more harm than good. Constant stress will also cause certain hormone levels (such as your cortisol) to be out of balance, which can cause health problems. Food can add stress to your body as well.

Stress also plays a huge role in our experience of pain. Stress can lead to headaches and other unpleasant symptoms. That said, it can be very difficult to live a stress-free lifestyle; the world is full of stressors, even putting aside those related to illness. However, if you take little steps to try to minimize your stress level every day, you will most likely see some decrease in your pain. Taking long walks outside (if you are up to it) can help you relax and let go of things. Meditation is another great way to let everything go; sometimes, we just need time to ourselves.

Samantha's Experience

If you asked my friends and family to name two of my top flaws, I am sure they would say I worry too much and do not know how to relax. However, in the last two years, I have slowly been working to let go of what I cannot change, because I know anxiety is harmful to my body.

One thing I have always loved doing is going to the beach; I find the sights and sounds to be very relaxing. I have also found listening to music allows me to unwind. I am able to forget about everything while rocking out to music (usually country music!). These are some ways I escape the world for a little while. Hopefully, they will help you to relax and stay calm, as well. I have also found that coloring can help relieve stress and have a calming effect.

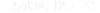

8

Related Illnesses

U NFORTUNATELY, OTHER illnesses can accompany endometriosis. In this chapter, I am going to touch a little on other pelvic pain conditions which may present with your endometriosis, but which you may not even know you're suffering from.

POLYCYSTIC OVARY SYNDROME (PCOS)
Polycystic ovary syndrome (PCOS) is a painful illness, and one which can lead to infertility. Many women who have endometriosis also have PCOS. It is a condition in which one or both ovaries are constantly covered with cysts, and it is caused by insulin resistance. Ovulation does not occur in those women who have PCOS and are not being treated for it.

PCOS is caused by imbalances in the workings of the body's endocrine system. The endocrine system is responsible for secreting hormones; if the endocrine system is not working right, the body's hormones will be out of sync. Medications can be used to treat this condition, which include metformin (also used for diabetics) and birth control pills. Pain and hair in unwanted places are common symptoms, as is infertility. (Note that even if a woman has a hysterectomy, she can still have disorders like polycystic ovary syndrome, because it is an endocrine disorder.)

There are many types of cysts that can form on a woman's ovaries. The most common are endometriomas (cysts that form from endometriosis), cystadenomas, and functional cysts. Ovarian cysts can be very painful and are caused by too much estrogen. They can either burst or be drained during surgery or an office visit by a doctor.

Many women have PCOS without even knowing it, which is unfortunate as, left undiagnosed, PCOS can lead to diabetes. Some women have also found that, with a diagnosis of PCOS, their insurance cost goes up, which is terrible. Women—or anyone, for that matter—should not have to worry about their insurance increasing because of a diagnosis. After all, a patient can only control their health up to a certain degree.

Samantha's Experience

My battle with PCOS is still ongoing, and I am sure that it will never go away entirely. My doctor increased my progesterone topical cream to 250mg twice daily, in addition to increasing my vitamin D intake to 5,000–10,000 units daily, which has helped. My headaches have gone away and my pain has decreased; however, I do still have some ovary and uterus pain.

I also started taking 500mg of metformin every day with dinner, though I did not notice anything different until the third day of treatment. On that day, I felt terrible; my doctor had warned me I might have an upset stomach, which I did, but I was still unprepared for the level of discomfort I experienced. I felt very nauseous, probably the most nauseous I have ever felt; I had a really bad headache, felt weak, and wanted nothing more than to lie in my bed until this feeling passed. I felt like this the entire day, but

> I managed to make it through, and even attended an interview for the pharmacy program.
>
> I called my doctor regarding the symptoms I was having from the metformin, and she recommended that I take half of a tablet (250mg) every day with dinner and see if that helped. And so far, so good; that dosage has worked for me, and I continued to take it until my hysterectomy.

ADENOMYOSIS

Adenomyosis is a condition in which the endometrium has penetrated and started to grow into the muscle layer of the uterus, which may cause heavy periods. It may be diagnosed during a pelvic exam, MRI, or ultrasound, depending on the doctor's expertise.

A great resource to learn more about adenomyosis is the article "What are the Indications for Hysterectomy?" from the Center for Endometriosis Care website[7].

VAGINISMUS

Vaginismus is a pelvic condition in which nothing is able to penetrate the vagina. In someone who is suffering from vaginismus, just the thought of anything penetrating (including a tampon) may be painful, and as a result penetration will not be able to occur. There is also a psychological component that may need to be addressed, as well. If you think you have this condition, talk to your doctor about being referred to a physical therapist for treatment to learn how to relax and change your thinking.

For more information on this and other pelvic pain conditions, *Stop Endometriosis and Pelvic Pain: What Every Woman*

---

7   http://centerforendo.com/what-are-the-indications-for-hysterectomy/

& Her Doctor Need to Know is a good resource. There is also a great book on stretching called *Heal Pelvic Pain* by Amy Stein. However, I recommend that you see a physical therapist first to get diagnosed with a pelvic floor condition, or else rule them out, before you start the stretches.

OVARIAN REMNANT SYNDROME

Ovarian remnant syndrome occurs when ovarian tissue is left over after the removal of both ovaries and fallopian tubes. The syndrome occurs when this ovarian tissue causes severe pelvic pain and/or a pelvic mass.

VULVODYNIA

Vulvodynia describes any chronic pain around the opening of the vagina that is otherwise unexplained.

PELVIC INFLAMMATORY DISEASE

This is a sexually transmitted disease that can cause pelvic pain.

OSTEOPOROSIS

Osteoporosis is a bone disease that occurs when the body loses too much bone, makes too little bone, or both. The bones become brittle and are more prone to break.

Osteoporosis is an illness that can accompany endometriosis. Women who are going through menopause are at an increased risk of having it because of a decreased level in estrogen, and osteoporosis occurs because of a low level of estrogen. Women who have tried Lupron as a treatment for endometriosis are said to be at an increased risk for osteoporosis because their bodies stop producing estrogen and go through a drug-induced menopause.

Samantha's Experience

Imagine my shock and dismay when my doctor called to tell me that I had osteoporosis at 24 years old.

When testing for osteoporosis, doctors will evaluate the average of your bone density at your femur, hips, and spine. A bone density that is lower than a score of -2.5 is considered osteoporosis. Mine was -3. My doctor also told me she was not yet sure what treatment to start me on because of my age. She did not want to put me on something long-term that would cause another issue down the road, and so referred me to an endocrinologist.

While on the one hand, I was thankful I'd insisted on having a bone scan done—it would have been worse to find out later and risk serious injury in the meantime—I was still incredibly upset. In fact, for days I could not stop crying. I really was 24 trapped in a 60-year-old's body. Even though I had done everything I could, I felt like my body was attacking itself. I did not know if I was going to be able to attend pharmacy school, or even if I'd be able to stay in my current apartment, which required me to walk up and down two flights of stairs each day. I simply had no idea what my quality of life would be from now on. I would have to be careful with everything I did, because I was now at a higher risk of breaking a bone.

I still do not know what caused it: low vitamin D, the hysterectomy, the three doses of Lupron I'd taken in the past, or a combination of all three. Neither did I know how long I'd had it, though I suspected it was to blame for a stress fracture I'd had three months prior.

Osteopenia

Osteopenia is a condition characterized by bone loss, but which has not yet reached the extent of true osteoporosis. In determining the extent of bone loss, doctors will use a rating called a "T-score." A T-score score is the measurement of how thick or dense human bones are. The more positive the measurement, the better; negative measurements are alarming and can signal health issues. The T-score for osteopenia is between -1 and -2.5. Many medical professionals do not like to use the word "osteopenia," so you may hear this also referred to as "low bone density."

Samantha's Experience

Prior to my appointment with the endocrinologist to discuss my back and knee pain, I read *Dr. Lani's No-Nonsense Bone Health Guide* so that I could be informed about osteoporosis and my treatment options. This allowed me to be more prepared for my appointment. It is important to have at least some idea of potential treatment plans, including which you agree with and which you do not want to try, before meeting with doctors to discuss your healthcare. That way, you don't end up going with the flow, talked into a treatment you don't agree with, or whose risks you don't fully understand (which is how I felt about agreeing to have Lupron injections).

As it turned out, I had many of the common risk factors for osteoporosis, including endometriosis, polycystic ovary syndrome, low body weight, vitamin D deficiency, hysterectomy (with both ovaries removed), early menopause, Caucasian ethnicity, past experience with Depo Provera and Lupron, and possible idiopathic scoliosis. Of note is the fact that most (if not all) of these risk factors are a direct result of my endometriosis and its treatment.

GASTROINTESTINAL ISSUES

Hormones can play a role in how our gastrointestinal system functions. Because of this, women with endometriosis often have gastrointestinal issues, as their hormones are not at the levels they should be for optimal health.

Irritable Bowel Syndrome

Irritable bowel syndrome is a disorder that may be incorrectly diagnosed in place of endometriosis because some of the symptoms are similar. Symptoms of irritable bowel syndrome (or IBS) include cramping, abdominal pain, bloating/gas, diarrhea, and constipation. It is typically diagnosed by having a colonoscopy. IBS does not cause inflammation or increase the chances of getting cancer.

Samantha's Experience

When my constipation and left side pain remained a problem, I went to my gynecologist, who suggested that I stop taking estrogen and focus on my gastrointestinal problems. If my left side pain decreased once I stopped the estrogen, she reasoned, this would mean that endometriosis was causing my pain. That said, she doubted that my past endometriosis had anything to do with my current pain. She did a pelvic exam to see if I had a yeast infection, which still hurt pretty badly, but I guess that is something I will always have to deal with.

Since I was still having difficulty emptying my bowels, I went to see a nurse practitioner. She listened to my heart and stomach as well as pushed on my abdomen. She said she could tell there was scar tissue in my abdomen because it crinkled when she pressed on it. I explained to her how constipated I was and that my left side hurt during bowel movements. She gave me Linzess samples to try, as well as a probiotic. She did not want to do a colonoscopy since I'd had one done four years ago, and it was unlikely I had a bowel obstruction.

I had bowel movements the first four days after I started taking Linzess, but on the fourth night, my left side started hurting badly. I had to take a pain pill and stay in the bed the next day. This was the same area the gastroenterologist had felt scar tissue. I was scared; what if it was the estrogen that was causing the pain? What if my back pain these past six months had been from constipation and not osteoporosis? More questions, without any firm answers.

My gastroenterologist scheduled me for a CT scan, the results of which came back the following week. Frustratingly, they showed that everything was normal. I could not understand this; I'd had to increase my Linzess dose from 145mg to 290mg and I was still only having a bowel movement every 1–2 weeks, which is not normal. It made me feel like the pain must all be in my head; after all, my doctors could not find the problem, even with all these tests.

A week after I stopped the estrogen, the amount of pain I was in made me feel like I was on my period. The following week (a week before I was due to have a colonoscopy), my pain had become unbearable, and worse yet, I had no idea why. I also had to take pain medication, which I really did not want to do because of my constipation issues.

The day before my colonoscopy, I was put on a strict clear liquid diet consisting of water, vitamin water, frozen fruit bars (like popsicles), and clear broth. At 5pm that day, I had to start the bowel prep, which consisted of Prepopik, a prescription I had to take several times with water. After midnight, I could no longer drink or eat anything until after my colonoscopy, which was scheduled for 2 PM the next day. This was probably the worst part: having to wait so long for the procedure without anything to eat. There were times when I felt like I was going to pass out or throw up, likely because I was dehydrated.

The colonoscopy itself only took about fifteen minutes and came back normal. The gastroenterologist told me to continue taking Amitiza for my constipation, along with a probiotic and stool softener. At this point, I was convinced my pain must be endometriosis-related because I had already tried Linzess and was now taking Amitiza. The question was, what was I to do now?

Gallbladder Complications

Estrogen can cause a gallbladder to become inflamed, which can lead to pain and possible gallstone formation. Testing can be performed to determine if a patient's gallbladder is functioning as it should and make the decision if the organ should be removed during a surgery called a cholecystectomy.

The gallbladder stores bile that is produced by the liver. When the bile duct is clogged, the gallbladder is unable to get bile out to the small intestine to help with digestion. There can be gastrointestinal issues that arise after having the gallbladder removed, so this should be discussed with your doctor before making your final decision. Symptoms of gallbladder issues include nausea, vomiting, pain where the gallbladder is located, and unusual stools.

Samantha's Experience

I called to schedule an appointment with my gynecologist to discuss my options. Because I was still having pain around my right ribs where my gallbladder is, we decided that I would have a HIDA (hepatobiliary) scan done to test how my gallbladder was functioning. I felt like my only option right now was surgery, believing that nothing else would help the pain. I also thought that I still had endometriosis, especially since my colonoscopy was normal.

We decided I would have surgery after my HIDA scan. If my gallbladder had to be removed, it could all be done in the same surgery by a general surgeon. If I was found to have endometriosis during this surgery, it would mean that the endometriosis specialist did not excise all of the disease. Since I had a hysterectomy, new implants could not form, but if all the disease was not removed it *can* continue growing.

The HIDA scan took an hour and a half and required me to remain lying still the whole time. The technician put an IV in my arm and injected it with a radioactive tracer so that my gallbladder, liver, and part of my bowels would show up. After an hour, a nurse came in and injected the IV with Kenevac, which would cause contractions in my gallbladder to see how it was functioning. When the Kenevac was injected, they warned me that my upper body pain might get worse, and to let them know if it did. Thankfully, the pain did not get worse.

My results from the HIDA scan were posted to my online portal the same day the test was done, and indicated that my "gallbladder ejection fraction" was low. A gallbladder ejection fraction is a measurement used to determine how well the gallbladder functions or empties. The higher the ejection fraction, the better the gallbladder is functioning. Mine was rated at 25 percent, with the normal range being 35 percent or higher.

I felt like the right thing to do at this point was to have my gallbladder removed, since it seemed to not be functioning properly and was causing me constant pain.

INTERSTITIAL CYSTITIS

Interstitial cystitis (sometimes called "painful bladder syndrome") is a very painful bladder condition marked by chronic bladder pressure, bladder pain, and pelvic pain. Many women who have endometriosis may be diagnosed with this first because it is easier for a doctor to diagnose. Other symptoms of this painful illness include incontinence, trouble emptying one's bladder, and painful urination.

There are several tests that can be done to see if you do or do not suffer from interstitial cystitis. These tests include an MRI and urinary testing to check your stream of urine. Your doctor may give you something to measure your urine and ask you to keep a diary for 24 hours to see how much water you are drinking versus how much you are urinating. Depending on those results, your doctor may decide to do a cystoscopy that will allow him or her to go in and see your bladder and take tissue samples for testing. Depending on how severe it is, your doctor may offer you different treatment options such as oral medications to help ease the pain.

If you think you have interstitial cystitis, or want to rule it out, ask your doctor about these testing options.

HEART DISEASE

Women who have endometriosis may also be at an increased risk for heart disease. This may be due to the rise in hysterectomies among women who have endometriosis, as researchers have found that surgical treatment of endometriosis—removal of the uterus or ovaries—may partly account for the increased risk of heart disease. It is important that women talk to their doctors about what they can do to decrease their risk of being diagnosed with heart disease, especially at a young age.

DEPRESSION

Many women who suffer with endometriosis also suffer with some form of depression because it can be difficult to cope with this disease. Not being able to do the things you were once able to do or the feeling of missing out on things because of your illness can be extremely depressing. It is important to talk to your doctor about any of these feelings you may have, and possibly think about getting a therapist if you think it could help you. Personally, it has helped me significantly.

There are medications your doctor can prescribe for depression if that is the direction you want to go in. Remember, you are not alone, and you will get through this one day at a time. The prevalence of suicides has become a topic of discussion because women feel there is no way out and no escape from the pain, which is heartbreaking. If you feel this way, please talk to someone. There are people who will listen to you and will try to help you find the answers that you are looking for.

There may be other illnesses associated with endometriosis that are not mentioned here. It is important for you to do research, as well, to make sure all of your bases are covered.

9

How Endometriosis Affects
Those Around Us

WHILE IT'S tempting to think otherwise, endometriosis affects more than just the person suffering with the illness. Although you are the only one in physical pain, those who love and care about you suffer with you. Of course, this is a two-way street; those around us also affect how we experience this illness. I've often felt like people look down on me or do not think I'm capable of something just because I am in pain. I cannot stand that; it makes me feel like I am not good enough to do what "normal" people do. Whenever I have to call in to work, I feel like they've lost faith in me each time. When I was off work, all I did was lie in bed because I was so tired. It was my parents, sister, extended family, friends, and co-workers who continued to help keep me going.

Speaking from personal experience, do *not* let go of those people who are willing to sit with you, watch movies with you, or be there for you in other ways. It is easy to respond to this amount of pain by self-isolating, and sometimes all you want is to be by yourself and cry. It's important to give yourself that kind of release, but having company can be a good thing.

It is so important that everyone in this situation feels they have a good support system. Without support and the added confidence it brings, we risk sliding further down into depression, which leads to more pain and misery. My family, who has seen me at my worst, has always been there for me.

> *Samantha's Experience*
> My family has been incredibly supportive throughout my entire fight with endometriosis. In addition to helping financially, they also rearranged their schedules so that at least one member of my family would be with me at each of my many doctors' appointments. Many nights, during especially bad flares, my mom would sleep with me in case I needed help. My mom and dad also went with me to all of my surgeries, whether they were local or out of town. They even took turns riding with me to my physical therapy appointments, which was about a six-hour round trip (my sister went with us if she was able to get time off from work).

Throughout this entire ordeal, I have tried to remain positive, despite the challenges involved. After all, it can be devastating to have to cancel plans with friends last-minute—not because you want to, but because you are in too much pain. It is even more devastating when they are rude to you for canceling, just because they do not understand how hard it is for you to get out of bed and do all of the things they take for granted—things like taking a shower, cooking, and working. But in the end, you have no choice but to remain positive, because the alternative is to remain trapped in your situation, never finding a way out, and never moving forward, which is an awful feeling.

MEDICAL EXPENSES

Medical expenses affect us as well as our families. Healthcare costs us so much; medical insurance is expensive, and on top of that, you usually must meet a deductible before your insurance will start covering anything. Not to mention, medical insurance can be a quagmire of red tape and restrictions, with no agreed-upon standard of coverage and inconsistent definitions of what constitutes a "medically necessary" procedure. For sufferers of endometriosis, a disease which is seemingly as difficult to diagnose as it is to treat, the financial burden of health insurance and repeated medical testing is all too familiar. Thankfully, it is possible to have payment plans set up before or after a procedure is done for patients who do not have health insurance or can't pay the full expense at one time.

Samantha's Experience

From 2010–2015, I had to switch insurance companies four different times. One of the insurance plans I was a dependent on was Obamacare. I personally had many issues with my coverage; there were only certain doctors who accepted my plan, which forced me to find new doctors. Once, when I'd found the doctor who agreed to do my hysterectomy, I learned that Obamacare would not cover an ultrasound that my doctor thought was medically necessary. However, because I was not pregnant (and would never *be* pregnant), the insurance company disagreed and refused to cover the cost, meaning I had to pay over $200 out of pocket. This ultrasound was done before my hysterectomy and showed that one of my fallopian tubes was swollen.

After Obamacare, I purchased coverage under

United Healthcare, which featured a $600 deductible for in-network doctors and $1200 deductible for out-of-network providers. However, the doctor that was going to do my fifth laparoscopic surgery wanted $4000 up front, because he was an out-of-network provider and I had not yet met my deductible. Without insurance, my fifth surgery would have cost me $50,000, between the hospital costs and all the different doctors who helped during my surgery. This is a ridiculous amount of money, and is a big part of why many people do not receive the healthcare they need. With my insurance, I had to pay a total of $5,000, which is still not cheap, especially since I had been unable to work. Still, I was thankful to not be responsible for paying the full amount.

10

Awareness

ENDOMETRIOSIS NEEDS so much more awareness than it currently has. Doctors and patients alike both need to be better equipped to handle endometriosis and its sufferers. The problem has causes on both sides: doctors require better, more accurate information to be available to them (and should have endometriosis covered more extensively in medical school curriculums); patients, on the other hand, need to do their own research on the treatment options available, regardless of whether they trust their doctor to present them with the best options. With the amount of misinformation currently in circulation, including confusing or conflicting medical studies, patients can no longer afford to simply accept what their doctor tells them. People do not understand endometriosis, even those who claim to be medical professionals.

There also need to be more widespread acceptance of the ill effects that endometriosis carries for those who suffer from it. I recall an interview with a celebrity doctor, in which he basically said that endometriosis is a diagnosis doctors give to women when they cannot figure out the real reason. He also went on to say that those women who *are* diagnosed with the disease must have been sexually abused, a misinformed and prejudiced statement so far from the truth it makes me sick to think of it. He has no idea what it is like to live in pain on a monthly or daily basis, or to sit and watch someone else suffer in excruciating pain. But sadly, his more extreme views aside, his level of ignorance is all too common, which is why the medical community responds to endometriosis the way it does.

WAYS TO RAISE AWARENESS

Endometriosis Walks

While there are currently endometriosis walks in Washington, D.C. and Hamilton, Waikato, New Zealand, there need to be more organized walks taking place the world over to help raise money to find a cure, as well as to raise awareness. The goal is to get people talking about endometriosis so that something can be done—sooner, rather than later.

The ROSE Study

The ROSE Study (Research OutSmarts Endometriosis) is a study that analyzes the medical history of patients with endo-metriosis, including surgery reports and their blood or saliva, to help determine the cause of endometriosis. Once you contact them, they will send you paperwork to complete regarding your medical history. They will then send you a blood or saliva kit for you to collect a sample and send back (the blood sample has to be collected by your doctor or lab; you can collect the saliva yourself). You can then choose to send all of your medical records to them or consent to have them contact your doctors to obtain the ones you want them to have. I chose to scan and email them all of my medical records because I felt that was easiest.

Social Networking

With the advent of social media, spreading the word and foster-ing community outreach is more efficient than ever. It is nice to know that there are other people who understand just how much pain you are really in, even though it is horrible to see so many people suffering with endometriosis. For example, there are really good Facebook support groups where you can post your story and get feedback from other endometriosis sufferers.

Some of the pages I have found are:

- Knock Out Endo

- Endometriosis Team

- Endometriosis Research Center

- Hormones Matter

- Hormone Soup

- ENDOVisible

- Endometriosis Awareness Campaign.

These are pages focused on helping women cope with endometriosis and find a cure. There are also many blogs out there that women have started to discuss their journey with endometriosis and hormones, as well as share relevant research to help those of us that suffer with endometriosis and raise awareness. If we all band together, we will not be ignored. It is time for us to make our voices loud and clear so that healthier treatment options and a cure will be found.

> **The Endo Buddy Program**
> Signing up for the Endo Buddy program (through the Endo Warriors group) is one of the best things I ever did. It's given me a chance to talk with someone around my age who is going through the same things I am. While I have a great support system in my family and friends, but they cannot fully understand what I've gone through, so talking with someone who can truly empathize has also helped me tremendously.

> My Endo Buddy and I have become very close in a
> short amount of time, because we understand—more
> than anyone else in our lives—what each other is
> going through. We talk to each other often, even if
> it's just to see how the other one is doing. (Unfortu-
> nately, we live a few hours apart, so we have only met
> face to face twice.)

Changes to Endometriosis Treatment

As I've stressed time and again throughout this book, one of the
most difficult parts of seeking relief from endometriosis are the
inadequacies in the care we receive from our current healthcare system. The difficulties of finding and retaining adequate
insurance; the struggle to find a competent, informed doctor
who will listen to what you have to say; and the challenges
inherent in conveying your symptoms to medical professionals
who either do not understand or will not believe you; it all
combines to create a never-ending obstacle course that would
exhaust a healthy person, much less someone in constant pain.
With that in mind, there are some changes I feel ought to be
made to how endometriosis is treated, based on my personal
experiences.

If a doctor wants to be a gynecologist, they should be required to learn about endometriosis, including the signs, symptoms, and available treatments. Furthermore, doctors should
work to make *every* patient feel like she has a say in deciding
which treatment is best for her. If the doctor is not open to
all treatments, he or she should be *required* to send the patient
to a medical professional who can better help them. Doctors
need to understand that it takes a team of medical professionals
working together to make a patient healthy; it should not be a
competition, beholden to market forces. I certainly would have

benefited had my first few doctors admitted they did not know what to do and sent me to a specialist.

Another alternative would be to only have endometriosis surgeons, or surgeons licensed to operate on endometriosis, operate on patients. Otherwise, mistakes will continue to be made by doctors who do not know what they are looking for. I also feel that it should be a requirement for all surgeons who perform surgery on endometriosis patients to send their biopsies to a research facility so that more research can be done to determine if there are better treatments out there and get closer to finding a cure.

Endometriosis and Disability

Endometriosis is a debilitating disease for most (if not all) women who suffer from it. It is hard for us to work when we are in so much pain and cannot find anything to relieve the pain. When a woman suffers from endometriosis, she is very limited as to what she can do and it is hard to stand for long periods of time. This is why I believe endometriosis should be recognized worldwide as a disability. That way, women with the disease would have some sort of income while they are not able to work, and can instead spend their time finding the answers they need regarding their health.

CONCLUSION

I'M NOW a couple months past my sixth surgery, which removed my gallbladder and some scar tissue from previous operations. While I've still had intermittent medical problems, on the whole my life is much improved, compared to where I was at the start of it all.

I am scheduled for a bone scan with my gynecologist in a couple of months to assess if my bone density has worsened, stayed the same, or improved since being on estrogen for more than a year. A bone scan done by my endocrinologist in November saw that my bone density has actually slightly improved. I am still using an estrogen patch, which I use once a week; I'm not confident enough to increase the amount of estrogen I take. I usually do not have headaches or hot flashes, and I still take 5000 units of vitamin D daily.

It has been difficult for me to find a doctor that will agree to prescribe bio-identical hormones for me, but since I know my body needs estrogen, I have been using the Climara patch in the interim until I can receive the proper prescription.

In terms of my quality of life, I no longer have lower back pain. I even went horseback riding, something I know I would not have been able to do if I still had my uterus and ovaries because of all of the bouncing. I had so much fun!

For a time, I was working full time (anywhere from eight to twelve hours, Monday through Friday) and spent many of my work hours standing. But in the end, this took too much of a toll on my body and resulted in pain and constipation issues. I took some time off to go to the doctor, but eventually decided to quit because I felt like it was the best decision for my body.

I have written about my life with endometriosis in the hopes that it will help people like me. I am telling my story because women with endometriosis should not have to have continuous surgeries in hopes of finding pain relief and living a "normal" life. When I think about endometriosis, I not only want to cry for myself, but for all of us who suffer with this debilitating disease.

I have high hopes that doctors all over the world will have this book in their waiting rooms for patients to read—that it will encourage patients to ask questions about their disease, which their doctors (hopefully) will be able to answer. Likewise, I want doctors to be more open to what their patients want.

When making decisions about your health, you need to be true to yourself. Do not let others influence your decisions— whether it is your parents, significant other, family, or friends trying to sway your decision. By no means am I telling you what to do, either. I am providing you with all of the treatment options I know about so that you can make a decision about which is best for your body. You have to do what is best for you, not what other people think is best for you.

And finally, remember that you do not know another person's story; it is not your place to judge. Just because you do not have a certain symptom of endometriosis that someone else does, does not mean either one of you are wrong. Everybody has different symptoms; you may both have the disease without suffering from the same symptoms. Everybody is different and experiences things differently.

I really hope all of this information helps you to get an answer about your pain sooner rather than later. I have enjoyed writing this book because I know it will help so many young girls and women gain better health, and it has served as an outlet for me to display my feelings, which has allowed me to relieve some stress.

I have learned just how strong I am because of having endometriosis. I've had to grow up fast and make decisions for myself that I should not have had to make, were it not for this disease. It takes a strong person to get out of bed every day knowing you are going to be in an extreme amount of pain. We are all fighters.

When I finish school, I want to do research on endometriosis so that I can try to help women suffering as I have, holding out hope of finding a cure. I will always strive to bring awareness to endometriosis however I can. This disease has left its mark on my life forever, and I am not going to stop fighting for us until we are heard.

—Samantha Bowick
Written July 2016-July 2017

MORE FROM THE AUTHOR

Hormones Matter is a website that educates people about different hormone issues as well as publishing personal stories of hormonal issues. After I saw a post on Facebook stating they were looking for writers, I decided to email them and received a response asking if I would like to tell my personal story with endometriosis. Since then, I have published a number of articles through Hormones Matter, sharing my experiences with those who are looking for help, hope, and answers. It continues to be important to me to write my story to let other women suffering with endometriosis know they are not alone, and to hopefully provide awareness for the disease.

My author page at Hormones Matter:
hormonesmatter.com/author/samantha-bowick/

My Battle with Endometriosis: Hysterectomy at 23
Published Jun 9, 2015
hormonesmatter.com/battle-endometriosis-hysterectomy-23/

How Do You Deal with the Lasting Effects of Endometriosis?
Published Sep 14, 2015
hormonesmatter.com/deal-lasting-effects-endometriosis/

Depression with Endometriosis
Published Dec 8, 2015
hormonesmatter.com/depression-endometriosis/

APPENDIX A:
WHAT TO BRING TO
A DOCTOR'S APPOINTMENT

The following is an example of what I take with me to any doctor appointment, to ensure that any new doctor I meet with has a full understanding and appreciation for the treatment avenues I've already explored. Note that I will also take with me the names of all the practitioners I've seen, which I have not included here. (It may also be helpful to download an app on your smartphone that will allow you to keep track of your periods so that you can tell your doctor if they are irregular, in addition to any symptoms you may be suffering. A food journal can also be a useful tool to determine if there are any underlying gastrointestinal issues.)

MEDICAL TIMELINE

Prescribed Ortho Tri Cyclen Lo (Tri-sprintec)

July 2010: Laproscopic surgery (cyst drained, endometriosis found)

2010–2011
   Received Lupron shot
   Prescribed Enjuvia 0.625 mg
   Depo shot
   Seasonique
   Prescribed Necon

December 2010: Received CT scan and colonoscopy
     Tested for Celiac disease (results negative)

January 2012: Laparoscopic surgery (cyst drained, no
     endometriosis)
     Prescribed Natazia

June 2012: MRI found fluid in pelvis–MUSC; tested for
     interstitial cystitis (results negative)

January 2013: Laproscopic surgery (hysteroscopy, cystoscopy,
     ureterolysis; cyst drained, endometriosis found)

April 2013: Received Lupron shot
     Prescribed Aygestin, Ovcon and Estrace
     Prescribed Progesterone Cream 40mg

May 2013: Was seen at Mayo Clinic in Jacksonville, FL
     Offered Prempro; refused
     Recommended pelvic floor physical therapy

June 2013: Began physical therapy for pelvic floor spasms

June 2013: Began gluten-free, dairy-free diet; continued for 2
     weeks
     Prescribed Progesterone 500mg bio-identical
     hormone cream and Metformin 250 mg for PCOS
     Prescribed magnesium 400mg for one month
     Taking liquid Vitamin D (5,000–10,000 units daily)

March 2014: Received hysterectomy, with bio-identical
     hormone treatment

March 2015: Laparoscopy surgery, removed endometriosis,
     nerves that connected to uterus, put bowels in correct
     location

February 2016: colonoscopy normal

April 2016: Gallbladder removed, scar tissue removed

September 2017: Estradiol patch 0.025mg
     Vitamin D 5,000 units daily (capsule)
     Polyethylene Glycol (Miralax) as needed

OTHER MEDICATIONS TRIED

- Ponstel 250 mg
- Ibuprofen 800 mg
- Cymbalta
- Celebrex 200 mg
- Toradol
- Tylenol 3
- Hydrocodone
- Tramadol 50 mg
- Percocet
- Spirinolactone
- Elavil
- Meloxicam

DIAGNOSES

- Vitamin D deficiency (2009)
- Endometriosis (July 2010)
- Irritable Bowel Syndrome (December 2010)
- Polycystic Ovary Syndrome (May 2013)
- Interstitial Cystitis (March 2015)
- Retroperitoneal Fibrosis (March 2015)
- Osteoporosis (July 2015)
- Curved spine/possible scoliosis (August 2015)
- Autoimmune disease; possibly fibromyalgia, arthritis (October 2015)

SURGERIES/PROCEDURES

- Tonsils and adenoids removed (1996)
- Tubes in and out of ears (1996)
- Laparoscopies
    + July 2010
    + January 2012
    + January 2013 (appendix removed)
    + March 2014 (hysterectomy; uterus, ovaries, and cervix removed)

+ March 2015
+ April 2016 (gallbladder removed)
- Colonoscopy (December 2011)
- Colonoscopy (February 2016)

APPENDIX B:
WHAT TO ASK YOUR
DOCTOR

No matter how many times you go to a doctor's office, it never stops being overwhelming. That's why it can be helpful to bring a list of general and specific questions with you to make sure that you get all the information you need.

The following is a sample list of basic questions I find helpful to ask any new doctor I see:

- What treatment options do I have for endometriosis to preserve my health and fertility as well as treat the pain and disease?
- Are there side effects to any of the treatments you're recommending?
- Will these treatments place me at a higher risk for other illnesses?
- What are the risks of surgery?
- What are the chances of my developing scar tissue a year or more after surgery?
- Do you work with other doctors or refer patients to specialists if there are bowel, gallbladder, gastrointestinal, etc. issues?
- If you are unsure how to treat my disease, can you refer me to an endometriosis specialist?

- Do you prescribe patients bio-identical hormones if they express interest in that treatment plan?
- How do you test hormone levels?
- Do you test for other illnesses, such as PCOS?

RESOURCES AND RELEVANT RESEARCH

ARTICLES & WEBSITES

The following is a list of articles and research studies related to endometriosis and its treatment that I feel are valuable in developing an understanding of your condition and the options available to you. By reading these articles, you empower yourself to make decisions as to the best route for your healthcare plan. I believe it is crucial that we all do our own research to understand the options we have as patients so we can better gauge what we think are the best treatment options for us.

"Endometriosis: Understanding a Complex Disease"
centerforendometriosiscare.com/understanding-endometriosis/

This is a comprehensive overview of endometriosis, presented by Dr. Ken Sinervo, one of the leading industry professionals in endometriosis treatment.

"Endometriosis In-Depth Report."
health.nytimes.com/health/guides/disease/endometriosis/print

This article offers a great description of what endometriosis is, where the disease can be found, and some theories on what causes it, as well as signs, symptoms, how to get diagnosed, and possible treatments to try to minimize pain.

"Mom's Endometriosis Means Increased Risk for Daughter."
www.womenshealthcaretopics.com/Blog/moms-endometri-
osis-means-increased-risk-for-daughter/
This article discusses the likelihood of a daughter having endometriosis when the mother has been diagnosed with the
disease.

"What is Endometriosis and What Are Your Choices" by Mar-
ilyn Glenville
www.marilynglenville.com/womens-health-issues/endome-
triosis/

In this article, the author discusses how essential it is that every
woman have their hormones balanced, as well as get the proper
balance of vitamins, minerals, and herbs, so that her body can
function at its optimum level. She goes on to discuss the types
of testing that can be done to test the blood levels of certain vitamins and minerals. Remember, it is important to discuss any
testing or supplements before you start taking them so your
doctor can better assist you.

"Pesticide exposure linked to increased endometriosis risk,"
Medical News Today
medicalnewstoday.com/articles/268399.php.

In this article, Medical News Today discusses the phenomenon
of whether pesticides increase the chance of a woman having endometriosis. One surprising statement is that "pesticides
raise endometriosis risk to 30–70%." The study mainly focused
on those pesticides that have estrogenic components, because
endometriosis is known to be the result of too much estrogen.

"Endometriosis Often Goes Ignored in Teenage Girls."
www.goodhousekeeping.com/health/news/a31956/en-
dometriosis-often-ignored/?src=spr_FBPAGE&spr_
id=1443_163588475

This article discusses how young girls who've just started their periods are brushed aside if they say they have endometriosis because doctors think there is no way they could have it at their age, when in reality they most likely do. Because of this misconception, girls/women do not trust doctors and go untreated, resulting in years of agonizing pain.

Peace with Endo
http://peacewithendo.com/2015/04/endometriosis-does-not-define-you.html.

Aubree Deimler wrote *From Pain to Peace with Endo* about her personal struggle with her disease; Peace with Endo is her blog. On this post on her blog, she shares her experience at the EndoMarch in Washington, D.C. and how women with endometriosis feel like burdens to their loved ones. Her book is great for those that want to try a natural approach instead of surgery. She also has a podcast called Peace with Endo that is free to listen to.

"The Natural Approach to Endometriosis: Getting to Your Root Causes"
avivaromm.com/endometriosis-natural-approach

Aviva Romm, MD is a doctor who uses natural remedies to help patients with endometriosis find a pain-free life without resorting to numerous surgeries. Her article discusses different supplements that can be added to one's diet to help reduce inflammation and help heal the body.

"Endometriosis is Often Ignored in Teenage Girls"
nytimes.com/blogs/well/2015/03/30/endometriosis-is-often-ignored-in-teenage-girls

Unfortunately, many medical professionals think that endometriosis is an adult woman's disease, which is not true. Adolescents show symptoms just as older women do. Because teenagers are not taken seriously by their doctors, the disease goes undiagnosed until years later. This can cause more problems since the disease has had more time to grow.

"What I Wish Everyone Knew About Endometriosis"
mindbodygreen.com/0-11318/what-i-wish-every-one-knew-about-endometriosis

This article by Libby Hopton discusses what endometriosis is and suggests that it is possible women are born with the disease, but do not show symptoms until after starting their period. She also lists ways women can try to change certain things in their lives to try to decrease pain if excision surgery is not an option.

"Women with endometriosis need support, not judgement"
medicalxpress.com/news/2015-03-women-endometriosis-judgement

This article discusses how expensive endometriosis can be and how the disease affects those that suffer with it. It is important that we have positive support from those around us to help us deal with these struggles. It is also important that we get people talking about the disease so that there is less negativity surrounding it.

"Drastic treatment for endometriosis after 20 years"
www.afr.com/lifestyle/health/womens-health/drastic-treatment-for-endometriosis-after-20-years-of-pain-20150324-1m5u3j

Written by Jill Margo, this is an article about a woman who went twenty years with endometriosis pain without getting much, if any, pain relief. In the article, the woman is said to have contemplated suicide because her pain was so horrible every month. She suffered with side effects of pain medications. However, most (if not all) pain medications are used for acute pain rather than chronic pain, which is why it is difficult to find pain medication that works for endometriosis pain.

"What Happens When Your Body Image Nightmare Comes True"
buzzfeed.com/virginiasolesmith/what-happens-when-your-body-image-nightmare-comes-true

Written by Virginia Sole-Smith, this is a great article about how women with endometriosis feel towards their bodies. Like the author, I know all too well what it is like to look in the mirror at my stomach and not like the scars I see or to not be able to wear what I want to because it does not fit appropriately. She discusses how upsetting it can be to be asked, "When are you due?" and ways she tries to be positive about her body. I think all women struggle with their appearance, but we should not. We are all uniquely different and beautiful.

"The Pain Test"
vox.com/2014/10/15/6895171/how-doctors-measure-pain-brain-scan-fmri.

"Doctors have no idea how much pain their patients are suffering. That's about to change." Written by Susannah Locke, is a very informative article about some changes that are taking place in healthcare. Dr. Sean Mackey is developing technology that will help doctors gauge the pain of each patient.

"I Could Have a Baby But She Could Not"
blitheblog.com/i-could-have-a-baby-but-she-could-not/
This is a blog written by a woman on the topic of infertility, and I think everyone should read it. She says, "What I've come to understand is that infertility is mostly a silent grief," which is very true.

"4 Huge Mistakes I Made During My Wife's Endo Battle"
www.braave.org/4-huge-mistakes-made-wifes-endo-battle/

This is an article written by a husband who feels like he failed his wife, who suffers with endometriosis, because he did not go to every appointment with her (among other things). I think it is hard for supporters because they may not understand what we are going through or how to help.

"Digesting it All!"
womensinternational.com/connections/digesting

This article discusses how the digestive system should be, including symptoms of gastric issues and how different hormones influence the GI tract. Some digestive diseases include: irritable bowel syndrome, Crohn's disease, ulcerative colitis, celiac disease, gallbladder disease, gastritis, gastroesophageal reflux disease, leaky gut syndrome, pancreatitis, and ulcers. This article also discusses how melatonin can help with irritable bowel syndrome symptoms.

"The Effect of Melatonin in the Treatment of Endometriosis"
drtorihudson.com/general/dietary-supplements/the-effect-of-melatonin-in-the-treatment-of-endometriosis/

Dr. Tori Hudson, a naturopathic physician, conducted a study to determine how taking 10mg of melatonin daily influenced women with endometriosis in Brazil. The study showed that the women who had the disease and took 10mg of melatonin every day had reduced pelvic pain. The placebo group did not see this change.

"Bloomin' Uterus: Suicide and Endometriosis"
bloominuterus.com/2014/12/23/suicide-endometriosis/

This article discusses the risk of suicide and suicide ideation in endometriosis patients, a heartbreaking truth.

"How can I manage my endometriosis-related pain?"
beyondbasicspt.wordpress.com/2015/03/17/how-can-i-manage-my-endometriosis-related-pain/

This article discusses different ways physical therapy can help decrease endometriosis pain.

"Endometriosis is an Autoimmune Disease"
larabriden.com/endometriosis-is-autoimmune/

This article suggests that endometriosis could be hormonal as well as autoimmune. This is partly because endometriosis has led to other diseases in females, such as irritable bowel syndrome. The author discusses things women with endometriosis might want to avoid, as well as things that may decrease symptoms.

"Why is my period late? You asked Google – here's the answer"
theguardian.com/commentisfree/2015/may/06/why-is-my-period-late-you-ask-google?CMP=fb_gu

This website discusses how much of a taboo it is to talk about menstruation, despite its being part of every woman's life, and therefore something that should not be viewed as disgusting. If we talked about it more, women would have a better understanding of their bodies and know what to look for.

"For women with endometriosis, answers are few"
washingtonpost.com/national/health-science/for-women-with-endometriosis-answers-are-few/

Darlena Cunha tells the stories of women with endometriosis and what doctors can do to help.

"How your sex life may influence endometriosis"
medicalxpress.com/news/2015-05-sex-life-endometriosis

This article discusses a study conducted by Dr. Jonathan Mc-Guane where endometriosis was found to increase when the disease comes in contact with seminal fluid. However, these findings have not yet been validated by real life subjects as of May 2015.

"5 Surprising Symptoms of Endometriosis"
prevention.com/health/symptoms-endometriosis

This article discusses five symptoms of endometriosis that may come as a shock to people. These include: gastrointestinal issues, upper body pain (including pain while breathing), infertility, frequent urination, and possible appendicitis.

"Hidden Clinical Trial Data about Lupron"
impactethics.ca/2014/05/02/hidden-clinical-trial-data-about-lupron

In this article, the author discusses the issues with Lupron, which can be a touchy subject between medical professionals and patients. She has spent decades trying to get the FDA to look into studies conducted on Lupron and accusations of fraudulent reporting on the injection. I strongly believe Lupron should not be on the market or pushed on endometriosis patients like it is, but that is just my opinion.

"High Rates of Gynecological Disorders Implicated in Chronic Fatigue Syndrome"
cortjohnson.org/blog/2015/05/06/

This blog discusses how gynecological disorders can lead to chronic fatigue. There were many statistics studied, but the one that stuck out to me the most is, "Women with [chronic fatigue syndrome] were four times more likely to have had a hysterectomy than women without it." This is especially apparent in women who were induced into menopause due to a hysterectomy years before the average age of menopause.

"Researchers shed new light on cause of Chronic Fatigue Syndrome"
https://medicalxpress.com/news/2015-05-chronic-fatigue-syndrome.html

This article discusses the research being done into chronic fatigue disorder, which I think is very relevant for those of us that suffer with endometriosis. It also discusses the signs and symptoms, which include "profound fatigue, muscle and joint pain, cerebral symptoms of impaired memory and concentration, impaired cardiovascular function, gut disorder, and sensory dysfunction."

"Why menopause won't cure endometriosis, fibroids, or ovarian cysts"
everydayhealth.com/news/why-menopause-wont-cure-endometriosis-fibroids-ovarian-cysts/

This is a very important article, because many of the doctors I have been to thought they could cure my pain by putting me on Lupron to medically induce menopause.

"Bloomin' Uterus: Library"
bloominuterus.com/library/

This is a list of endometriosis books you can borrow to read from another Endo sister.

"10 Signs It's Time To Dump Your Doc"
prevention.com/health/healthy-living/signs-you-need-new-doctor

This article lists warning signs as to whether your doctor is providing the standard of care you need. If your doctor displays any one of these signs, my recommendation is to find another one.

"Nonsurgical, quick and accurate test for diagnosing endometriosis discovered"
news-medical.net/news/20090819

This is an article published in 2009 about a nonsurgical way to diagnose endometriosis in Australia, Belgium, and Jordan. A device is inserted into the vagina to test if there are nerve fibers, which will tell if endometriosis is present. This would be awesome to have everywhere, especially if it is accurate.

"Global Consortium Identifies Best Management of Endometriosis"
nichd.nih.gov/news/resources/spotlight/Pages/041013-endometriosis

This article discusses different treatment plans for different groups for endometriosis patients, including adolescents, pregnancy, menopause, medical management of pain, and complementary therapies for pain.

"Endometriosis and MTHFR: A Connection"
mthfr.net/endometriosis-mthfr/2012/03/24/

This article discusses a possible link between genes and the environment on endometriosis.

"Facts About Endometriosis and Filing for Disability"
http://www.ssdrc.com/ssd-endometriosis.html

This is how to file for social security disability with endometriosis, but it is hard to get approved.

"Endometriosis treatment is 'unacceptable' and women are being failed"
glamourmagazine.co.uk/features/health-fitness/2015/endometriosis-symptoms-back-pain-during-pregnancy-period

This article discusses what endometriosis is, how important it is to seek help if you have any symptoms, and the possibility of the disease being autoimmune. It is important for patients to know what to ask doctors because unfortunately, many doctors will not offer a lot of information without being asked.

"Deep Excision Surgery, the Gold Standard of Endometriosis Treatment and Finding Endometriosis Excision Specialist"
drseckin.com/surgical-excision-for-endometriosis-the-gold-standard

This article discusses how surgery should be performed to remove all endometriosis. What I especially like about this article is the statement, "No surgeon should attempt endometriosis laparoscopic surgery if they have not mastered suturing techniques for bowel and bladder repair." I feel this is so important for doctors to realize, because the disease can be anywhere and they need to be equipped to handle every scenario; if they are not, they need to send their patient to a doctor who is.

"Endometriosis and Women's Health"
articles.mercola.com/sites/articles/archive/2004/09/29/endometriosis-health

In this article, Dr. Carolyn Dean discusses what endometriosis is, what the symptoms of the disease are, reasons to have saliva testing done, and supplements you can try to relieve some of your pain. I wish I would have come across this article when I first started having problems.

"Curcumin inhibits endometriosis endometrial cells by reducing estradiol production"
ncbi.nlm.nih.gov/pmc/articles/PMC3941414

This article discusses how curcumin could possibly inhibit endometriosis cells. Curcumin is a naturally occurring phytochemical and an extract of turmeric.

"What it Really Means to Have Endometriosis"
vitalhealth.com/blog/what-it-really-means-to-have-endometriosis/

Dr. Cook, a well-known endometriosis specialist, writes about what it is like to live with the disease.

"Researchers Find Link Between Endometriosis And Bone Deterioration"
nytimes.com/1988/03/08/science/researchers-find-link-between-endometriosis-and-bone-deterioration

This article discusses the possible link between endometriosis and bone loss. Interleukin-1 is a hormone that is found in women who have endometriosis and can interfere with bone growth. In my opinion, it is definitely worth having your doctor do a bone density scan to make sure your bones are as thick and healthy as they need to be.

"Toxic Link to Endo"
endometriosisassn.org/environment

This article discusses how toxic chemicals can affect endometriosis, including dioxin, which can be found in things that contain chlorine, like PVC plastic.

"Decreased Endometriosis Risk Associated with Strenuous Exercise"
womenfitness.net/decreased_endometriosis

This article discusses how exercise can decrease the amount of endometriosis by decreasing estrogen. However, since endometriosis pain can often inhibit one's ability to get up, get out, and exercise, it's not a perfect solution.

"New treatment for endometriosis preserves fertility"
newscientist.com/article/dn26892-new-treatment-for-endo-metriosis-preserves-fertility/

This article discusses two possible treatments for endometriosis that most likely do not cause infertility, using the drugs chloroindazole and oxabicycloheptene sulfonate. This may lead to women not having to choose to have surgery, though more research needs to be done on both drugs.

"Endometriosis: Devastating for Young Women"
huffingtonpost.com/erin-havel/endometriosis-devastating_b_5614112

This is a very informative interview between a woman whose friend has endometriosis and an endometriosis specialist—Dr. Eric Heegaard from Minneapolis, a noted advocate for endometriosis awareness.

"Seven reasons why Endo-Fatigue causes so much trauma to its sufferers"
survivingendometriosis.com/2014/11/25
Endo fatigue is very real and makes daily tasks harder to accomplish. This article discusses reasons why it is hard to live with.

"The Spoon Theory"
butyoudontlooksick.com/wpress/articles/written-by-christine/the-spoon-theory/

The "Spoon Theory" is a great way to explain to family and friends how you feel on a daily basis struggling with endometriosis.

"ASRM2015: Endometriosis may infiltrate the entire body" endometriosis.org/news/congress-highlights/asrm2015-endometriosis-may-infiltrate-the-entire-body/

Medical professionals at Yale University have been researching endometriosis to get closer to finding a cure. Professor Hugh Taylor has found that the most common form of endometriosis is peritoneal endometriosis, but the disease can be found anywhere and has many types.

"Ovarian Remnant Syndrome" centerforendometriosiscare.com/ovarian-remnant-syndrome-by-dr-ken-sinervo

This is an article written by Dr. Ken Sinervo, who graciously provided the foreword to this book, describing ovarian remnant syndrome and how to test for it.

BOOKS
The *Endo Patient's Survival Guide to Endometriosis & Chronic Pelvic Pain* by Dr. Andrew Cook, MD FACOG and Libby Hopton MS
This is a book that illustrates endometriosis in a straightforward and educational way, and is geared towards both patients and their loved ones. Dr. Cook is an endometriosis specialist practicing in California, and Libby Hopton works at his office.

The Doctor Will See You Now by Dr. Tamer Seckin
This is a great book to read to learn more about endometriosis. Dr. Seckin is an endometriosis specialist located in New York

who helped found the Endometriosis Foundation of America.

Fighting Fiercely: Unveiling the Unknown about Endometriosis by Michelle N. Johnson
This is a book about a woman's journey with endometriosis. She also has a website: www.fightingfiercely.com.

Alone in the Crowd: Living Well with Endometriosis by Ania G.
This is a book about a woman's life living with endometriosis and some changes she has made to help minimize her pain.

Endopocalypse: It Won't Kill You, But It Will Make You Wish You Were Dead by Nicole Jones
This is a book about one woman's life with endometriosis.

Heal Endometriosis Naturally: WITHOUT Painkillers, Drugs, or Surgeries by Wendy Laidlaw
This is a book about a woman's healing journey with endometriosis.

VIDEO
Endo What?
endowhat.com
This is a documentary that helps women and loved ones understand endometriosis, as well as spread awareness about the disease.

OTHER RESOURCES
The following are additional resources that may be valuable to those looking to expand their understanding of endometriosis and their treatment options. This is not a comprehensive list of every endometriosis resource or personal story that is available, but as I've stressed throughout this book, it is important to make sure you are well-informed and up-to-date.

Endometriosis: The Complete Reference of Taking Charge of Your Health
Written by Mary Lou Ballweg and The Endometriosis Association
This title has also been translated into Spanish.

The Endometriosis Sourcebook
Written by Mary Lou Ballweg and The Endometriosis Association

My Fem Truth: Scandalous Survival Stories
Written by Silvia Sidney Young

The Endometriosis Health and Diet Program: Get Your Life Back
Written by Dr. Andrew Cook

ABOUT THE AUTHOR

S AMANTHA BOWICK is from South Carolina, where she attended the University of South Carolina-Aiken for two years, taking pre-pharmacy courses in hopes of attending pharmacy school, until her endometriosis made that impossible. She then attended Columbia Southern University online and received a Bachelor of Science degree in Healthcare Administration, and received a Master's degree in Public Health from Liberty University online. She hopes to use her education and experiences to help women who suffer with endometriosis.

Connect with Samantha on social media!
Facebook: Samantha Bowick
Twitter/Instagram: @skbowick